Building Preverbal Communication & Engagement

Building Preverbal Communication & Engagement

Triadic Gaze Intervention for Young Children With Disabilities and Their Families

by

Lesley B. Olswang, Ph.D., CCC-SLP
University of Washington
Seattle

Julie L. Feuerstein, Ph.D., CCC-SLP
University of Central Florida
Orlando

and

Gay Lloyd Pinder, Ph.D., CCC-SLP, C/NDT
Children's Therapy Center
Kent, Washington

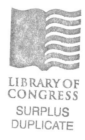
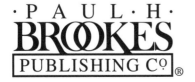

·P A U L·H·
BROOKES
PUBLISHING CO.®

Baltimore • London • Sydney

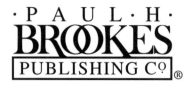

Paul H. Brookes Publishing Co.
Post Office Box 10624
Baltimore, Maryland 21285-0624
USA

www.brookespublishing.com

Typeset by Absolute Service Inc., Towson, Maryland.
Manufactured in the United States of America by Versa Press, Inc.

Library of Congress Cataloging-in-Publication Data
Names: Olswang, Lesley B., author. | Feuerstein, Julie, L., author. | Pinder,
    Gay Lloyd, author.
Title: Building preverbal communication & engagement: Triadic Gaze
Intervention for young children with disabilities and their families /
    by Lesley B. Olswang, Ph.D., CCC-SLP, Julie L. Feuerstein, Ph.D., CCC-SLP,
    and Gay Lloyd Pinder, Ph.D., CCC-SLP, C/NDT.
Description: Baltimore, Maryland: Paul H. Brookes Publishing Co., 2022. |
    Includes bibliographical references and index.
Identifiers: LCCN 2021023521 (print) | LCCN 2021023522 (ebook) | ISBN
    9781681254661 (paperback) | ISBN 9781681254685 (epub) | ISBN
    9781681254678 (pdf)
Subjects: LCSH: Communicative disorders in children. |
    Communication—Social aspects. | Speech therapists—Practice. | BISAC:
    EDUCATION / Special Education / Communicative Disorders | EDUCATION /
    Special Education / Developmental & Intellectual Disabilities
Classification: LCC RJ496.C67 O47 2022 (print) | LCC RJ496.C67 (ebook) |
    DDC 618.97/6855—dc23
LC record available at https://lccn.loc.gov/2021023521
LC ebook record available at https://lccn.loc.gov/2021023522

British Library Cataloguing in Publication data are available from the British Library.

2025   2024   2023   2022   2021

10   9   8   7   6   5   4   3   2   1

Contents

About the Video Clips and Downloads

Purchasers of this book can access the illustrative video clips for Chapters 1, 6, and 7 and Appendix C, which demonstrate the Triadic Gaze Intervention protocol, by streaming them from the Brookes Download Hub:

- Chapter 1: Video 1.1, a montage illustrating babies' typical development of preverbal communication behaviors

- Chapter 6: Videos 6.1–6.18, brief clips showing child and adult communication behaviors that illustrate discrete aspects of the Triadic Gaze Intervention protocol

- Chapter 7: Video 7.1 showing a practitioner working with a father to help him support his son's communication and engagement

- Appendix C: Videos 1–3 illustrating use of Triadic Gaze Intervention with three children with varied strengths, challenges, and support needs

Purchasers may also download, print, and/or photocopy the communication checklists and other provided resources for professional use.

To access the materials that come with this book:

1. Go to the Brookes Download Hub: http://downloads.brookespublishing.com

2. Register to create an account (or log in with an existing account).

3. Redeem the code **HovoLjUEK** to access any locked materials.

About the Authors

Lesley B. Olswang, Ph.D., Professor Emeritus, Department of Speech and Hearing Sciences at the University of Washington, Seattle

Dr. Olswang's 40-year tenure at the University of Washington included a professorial appointment in the Department of Speech and Hearing Science and a research affiliate appointment at the Center on Human Development and Disability. She received her academic degrees at Northwestern University, the University of Illinois, and the University of Washington. Dr. Olswang's honors include the University of Washington Distinguished Teaching Award and the Marsha Landolt Distinguished Graduate Mentor Award, a Fulbright Scholar's Award to study in the United Kingdom, Fellow and Honors of the American Speech-Language-Hearing Association, and Editors Awards from *Language, Speech and Hearing Services in Schools* and the *American Journal of Speech Language Pathology.* Dr. Olswang has had extensive clinical and research experience with children with language disorders. Her first clinical experiences involved developing a screening program for preschoolers in Evanston, Illinois, as the U.S. Education for All Act (PL 108-446) was initially being implemented. Her clinical research career has focused on two primary groups of children with communication challenges: school-age children and children below the age of 3. Her school-age research has examined the social communication of children diagnosed with fetal alcohol syndrome as they participate in classroom activities. Her research with children below the age of 3 has focused on two specific populations: toddlers diagnosed with specific language impairment and infants diagnosed with moderate to severe disabilities. She has been investigating the efficacy of treatment with these children and their families, particularly attempting to determine readiness factors for predicting benefits from different intervention options. Her primary research efforts in the last several years have been investigating the efficacy and implementation of Triadic Gaze Intervention, which was designed to assess and teach gaze shift as an intentional signal of communication to very young children with disabilities and complex communication needs. This research has been dedicated to improving the engagement and communication between children and their families as they encounter the struggles associated with disabilities. Dr. Olswang's research has been supported by grants from the University of Washington, The Arc of Washington State, the U.S. Department of Education, the National Institutes of Health, and the Centers for Disease Control.

Julie L. Feuerstein, Ph.D., CCC-SLP, Assistant Professor, School of Communication Sciences and Disorders, University of Central Florida, Orlando

Dr. Feuerstein is an Assistant Professor at the School of Communication Sciences and Disorders at the University of Central Florida. She obtained her master's degree in speech-language pathology at Boston University and her doctorate in communication sciences and disorders at the University of Washington. She completed postdoctoral training in the Department of Psychiatry and Behavioral Sciences at the Johns Hopkins School of Medicine, with an appointment to Kennedy Krieger Institute's Center for Autism and Related Disorders. Dr. Feuerstein is a certified speech-language pathologist who has practiced in a variety of pediatric practice settings, including early intervention, outpatient clinics, and inpatient rehabilitation. She is a member of the American Speech-Language Hearing Association, Neuro-developmental Treatment Association, International Society for Augmentative and Alternative Communication, and Society for Implementation Research Collaboration. Dr. Feuerstein's research interests center around evaluating the effectiveness of early communication interventions for minimally verbal children with neurodevelopmental disorders and examining mechanisms for moving empirically supported interventions into clinical practice. Her pre- and postdoctoral research has been supported by research awards from the American Speech-Language-Hearing Foundation, the University of Washington, and Kennedy Krieger Institute's Center for Autism and Related Disorders and by institutional training grants from the National Institutes of Health.

Gay Lloyd Pinder, Ph.D., Founder and past Therapist at Children's Therapy Center in Kent, Washington, and a Certified Neurodevelopmental Treatment (NDT) Speech Instructor

Dr. Pinder is a speech-language pathologist who has specialized for the past 45 years in working with infants and children with neuromuscular disorders and oral motor/feeding and communication problems associated with those disorders. Dr. Pinder received her academic degrees from Hollins University, Boston University, and the University of Washington. Dr. Pinder is a founder and continues to consult at Children's Therapy Center in Kent, Washington, a neuromuscular center serving children birth to 18 and their families. She is a certified NDT instructor and teaches courses in the United States as well as internationally. She has also been an instructor at the University of Washington in the Department of Speech and Hearing Sciences. Dr. Pinder's awards include the University of Washington Distinguished Alumna award; Duncan Award for exceptional service for children with disabilities, their families, and their communities; Washington Speech and Hearing Association Award for Clinical Achievement; and the Neuro-Developmental Treatment Association Award of Excellence. Dr. Pinder's therapy is child centered and family focused and is based on a holistic perspective of development. Dr. Pinder is a member of the American Speech-Language-Hearing Association; Washington Speech, Language and Hearing Association; National Association of the Deaf; and the Neuro-Developmental Treatment Association. Dr. Pinder's research has focused on the development of early communication signals in young children with neuromuscular disorders and then on treatment efficacy in teaching those early signals to those same children. She has also worked on research projects focused on training parents and most recently on training clinicians working in homes with that same population.

Preface

This book is the product of over three decades of research and clinical work with children and families who experience the challenges of moderate to severe disabilities that interfere with engagement and communication. The book is based on our deep belief that these children have a drive to connect with others and that early support services are responsible for giving them and their families a way to successfully start and succeed in doing so. The content of this book describes an intervention that serves as a guide for building children's capacity to communicate through preverbal behaviors. This capacity becomes the foundation for connecting with others and is the first step to successful interactions and future learning.

The power of communication early in life is breathtaking: A child's shared gaze with a caregiver, making sounds to express joy while looking at an adult, or reaching for a desired toy, are just some examples of the powerful behaviors that entice caregivers to engage with their young children. Caregiver–child engagement and communication during the first year of life lay the foundation for later learning across developmental domains. The importance of adult–child connections and interactions cannot be minimized. Yet, for many children, successful engagement and communication is hindered by motor, sensory, cognitive, and/or social impairments (e.g., children with cerebral palsy, congenital conditions, genetic syndromes, autism). The resulting disruption in adult–child interactions can threaten the joy of engagement and communication, and even future development. Triadic Gaze Intervention (TGI) was developed in the 1990s to address these challenges. It is an evidence-based intervention based on literature investigating typical development, which demonstrates the value of gaze behavior, along with gestures and vocalizations, as signals of early communication. From this literature, TGI was designed to encourage connections and interactions between children with disabilities and their communication partners. It is a strategy to be used in birth-to-three services that was developed to build children's preverbal behaviors of gaze, gestures, and vocalizations, culminating in intentional productions to enhance successful engagement and communication early in life. TGI should be viewed as a strategy that is practical and easily adaptable to a variety of children with disabilities and their families.

This book is designed to provide birth-to-three practitioners with a practical guide for working directly with caregivers. Professionals who serve this population, including speech-language pathologists, occupational therapists, physical therapists, and educators, will be guided through TGI as a conceptual strategy for facilitating engagement and early preverbal communication. TGI is implemented through a six-element protocol known by the acronym *PoWRRS-Connect* (providing opportunity, waiting, recognizing, responding, shaping, and connecting). This protocol is designed to increase children's productions of recognizable early preverbal communication signals within everyday activities and routines. It is a protocol that targets the production of behaviors that indicate intentional communication. Essentially, TGI and the PoWRRS-Connect protocol fit into mandated birth-to-three services and procedures that are used throughout the United States with children with a variety of developmental disabilities. Because practitioners provide services in natural environments, they are required to come up with strategies that caregivers can use to address concerns related to individualized family service plan (IFSP) goals. TGI can be one of those strategies. TGI embraces the significance of early engagement and communication by focusing on building skills that are necessary for successful interactions with others. The PoWRRS-Connect protocol used to deliver TGI is easily learned and will give practitioners a tool that can be utilized with a variety of young children and their families as they address a range of different IFSP goals. Our hope is twofold: First, we hope that early engagement and communication is considered a priority in birth-to-three services for children with disabilities that inhibit their connections with people and objects in their world. Second, we hope TGI and the PoWRRS-Connect protocol will be a valuable resource for practitioners as they provide services to facilitate intentional communication between children and others.

This book is written for practitioners who work with infants and toddlers, and their families. However, over the many years conducting TGI research with families and practitioners, and across our experiences presenting this work at local and national conferences, we have found that many of the techniques described in the PoWRRS-Connect protocol apply to individuals with developmental disabilities who may be well beyond the birth-to-three age range but find themselves in the early stages of communication development. We encourage practitioners to explore the utility of the PoWRRS-Connect protocol with clients and families who may benefit from a focus on early communication and engagement, regardless of their chronological age.

This book is organized into three sections. Section I provides information that describes early communication development and an overview of TGI. Chapter 1 provides background information describing typical early engagement during the first year of life and behaviors that signal communication with others. This background highlights the importance of gaze as an early signal of communication and demonstrates the significance of triadic gaze as a pivotal behavior in becoming an intentional communicator. The significance of this behavior, in turn, shaped the name Triadic Gaze Intervention. For children with moderate to severe disabilities, the development of these early communication behaviors is often seriously disrupted. Chapter 2 defines this population of children and highlights the challenges they face during social interactions. The chapter also includes a brief overview of effective interventions, along with a description of TGI and the research evidence supporting it. Chapter 3 discusses TGI in the context of the evolution of birth-to-three services in the United States since its inception, describing how TGI fits into mandated procedures.

From this background information, Section II describes TGI as the conceptual strategy and the PoWRRS-Connect protocol as a tool through which to implement TGI into birth-to-three services. The section starts with Chapter 4, an introduction to the purpose of TGI; who should deliver the PoWRRS-Connect protocol; and where, when, and why the protocol should be delivered. This chapter also presents an overview of the six basic elements that comprise PoWRRS-Connect: providing opportunity, waiting, recognizing, responding, shaping, and connecting. Chapters 5, 6, and 7 go into the details of TGI and PoWRRS-Connect, including, respectively, how to evaluate and assess the appropriateness of the TGI strategy for children and families, how to deliver the six basic elements of the PoWRRS-Connect protocol with the purpose of increasing children's recognizable communication behaviors, and how to implement the protocol with families during everyday routines. Chapter 8 offers suggestions for tailoring the implementation of TGI and PoWRRS-Connect with individual families and children. These tips, based on years of experience with TGI, are meant to provide practical ideas to practitioners as they work with families and children with a range of disabilities and characteristics. Chapter 9 offers suggestions for monitoring progress regarding engagement and communication, to address incremental changes that contribute to IFSP goals.

The final section of the book consists of one chapter, Chapter 10, which begins to address the complicated and varied journeys of young children with moderate to severe disabilities as they become older and adopt different ways to communicate. This chapter is different from the others. It consists of four stories from mothers of children with complex communication needs who were asked to reflect on their journey with early support services and describe their children's current communication. The mothers' reflections capture the potential of TGI for building a foundation of preverbal behaviors that led to successful, intentional engagement and communication with their children. The stories also reveal the various paths the children have taken in communication, culminating with the take-home message: "All children will learn to communicate, no matter the form, and engage with their world."

Throughout the book, we have provided numerous video examples to illustrate various aspects of the content we are describing. We hope these videos will clarify details regarding the administration of the PoWRRS-Connect protocol and demonstrate how easily it can be implemented in families' daily routines. We are mindful that successful service delivery for young children with disabilities is based on a strong partnership between practitioners and families. With this in mind, we have provided practitioners with handouts for caregivers describing early communication and PoWRRS-Connect in the appendices and on the Brookes web site for easy access. We encourage practitioners to use them freely and share the video examples when partnering with families.

Our journey to this book has covered more than 30 years; the work has been extraordinarily exciting as we have watched young children with extreme challenges move from limited and frustrating communication efforts to successful connection with their families and their worlds through TGI. As we struggle with the pandemic of 2020 that has struck the world, we consider the enormous challenges facing families of children with disabilities. This crisis has made us only more committed to our efforts to work with these children and their families, providing them with the best services to support their early developmental journeys. We strongly believe that the information presented in this book will improve engagement and communication between children with disabilities and their families. We further believe that TGI can be implemented through a variety of service delivery models, from in-person to telehealth, and become a powerful strategy for practitioners who support infants and toddlers. With pleasure and excitement, we offer this book and welcome you to join us in the TGI journey.

HAVE FUN!

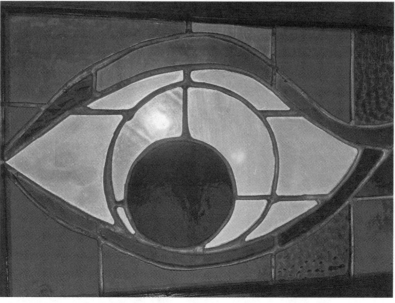

"The Eyes Have It" stained glass artwork by Becca Hanson, TGI team member.

Foreword

When PL 99-457 was enacted in 1986, Congress recognized the importance of early intervention to enhance the development of infants and toddlers with disabilities and to strengthen the capacity of families to meet the special needs of their infants and toddlers with disabilities. This law, now Part C of the Individuals with Disabilities Education Act (PL 108-446), ensures that young children with disabilities or at risk for disabilities and their families have access to supports and assistance through early intervention systems. Although some young children with disabilities received therapeutic and education services prior to this law, access often depended on the child's diagnosis or simple geography—services were not widespread. The law jump-started an exciting period that involved establishing new services and systems. It also spurred much research into identifying effective intervention practices and understanding how to shape those practices so that they are useful and acceptable for families.

This book builds on a strong evidence base, including a decades-long program of research conducted by the authors. The evidence base is coupled with the professional knowledge the authors have acquired through their real experiences with children, families, services, service providers, and policies. The research evidence and experience are complemented with a clear conviction for providing the highest quality supports that truly make a difference for children and families.

Some accounts of effective early intervention practices lack the specificity that is required to address the needs of very young children with moderate and severe disabilities and complex communication needs. This book focuses on those children and their families during that period of time when most children and families are delighting in the wonder of the back-and-forth interactions between baby and caregiver. For some children and their families, those wonderful interactions do not happen without support. *Building Preverbal Communication & Engagement* focuses on what happens when those interactions are disrupted and how to intervene to achieve smoother, more balanced interactions and engagement that make possible communication and learning.

It is now almost commonplace to write that development and learning occur within the context of relationships. As the authors write, the fundamental element of relationships is the back-and-forth exchange or turn-taking that sets the stage for learning. Long before words or conventional communication, caregivers interpret the baby's gaze, gurgles, and gestures as having meaning. Caregivers respond and add to the exchange. But sometimes, notably when the child has some sort of significant disability, it can be difficult to see or read the child's signals. Caregivers can become frustrated. Families are sometimes at a loss. Interactions break down. Relationships can flounder. Practitioners can also be challenged. They have learned about the importance of relationships. Engaging in the serve and return of early interactions seemed so straightforward when they were reading their textbooks, but the practitioner's frustration can grow when the child assumes unusual postures, grimaces, or seems to make very little progress.

This is where *Building Preverbal Communication & Engagement*—and specifically Triadic Gaze Intervention (TGI)—fills an important gap. This set of intervention practices, operationalized into six steps, is designed for very young children with significant disabilities and their families to meet the needs and challenges of engaging and communicating with each other. It aims to help caregivers and children become increasingly skilled at reading and responding to each other, even when the child's earliest attempts are very difficult or seemingly impossible to recognize and interpret. TGI provides detailed guidance for achieving successful adult–child interactions. TGI places the intervention in the context of natural, daily routines that make up the fabric of family life. At the same time, the approach appreciates the realities of everyday life and caregiving responsibilities. Thus, the authors offer options and modifications to better fit a family's preferences and styles.

However, this book is not just about a set of evidence-based intervention practices, valuable as that is. The book aims to help practitioners, speech-language pathologists, and other early interventionists gain the knowledge and skills they need to partner with and coach families to use the practices. The approach helps practitioners think about the diversity of families and family life and how to support families in making their own decisions about the routines and activities, times, and places that make sense for them. Once again, the guidance for practitioners is based on research. The authors undertook not just efficacy studies but also implementation studies. Practitioners will benefit from an evidence-based approach that appreciates the nuances of how effective early intervention can be delivered.

The intervention practices described in this book align with the American Speech-Language-Hearing Association's guiding principles in early intervention as well as Part C requirements. Furthermore, the practices correspond with the Division for Early Childhood's Recommended Practices. Thus, the practices represent the collaboration and cross-disciplinary knowledge and practice that is so important for effective early intervention.

The authors draw from their combined experiences as researchers, talented clinicians, and teachers who have prepared speech-language pathologists and other practitioners to develop the expertise to fulfill their early intervention responsibilities. This highly readable book offers readers the developmental and research background that establishes both the importance and substance of TGI. The authors carefully describe the intervention protocol (PoWRRS-Connect—provide opportunity, wait, recognize, respond, shape, connect). They help readers understand how TGI fits within the Part C steps, procedures, and service delivery guidelines. Readers will learn how to monitor child progress toward triadic gaze and how to link with tracking progress on IFSP goals. The authors spend considerable time describing how to put the TGI practices into action with families and how to adjust the intervention to better respond to individual family situations and preferences.

The book focuses on the earliest years and spotlights all that it takes to accomplish triadic gaze for some children and families. The final chapter will help readers appreciate how important this milestone is by telling the stories of four families who have participated in TGI. The mothers reflect on their early frustrations with how difficult it was to interact with their young child, what the intervention practices and the support from a skilled and compassionate practitioner meant to them, and where they and their children are today. In fact, throughout the chapters, the text is enriched with vignettes, stories, and quotes that bring the approach to life. These are not just single examples but multiple examples that recognize the uniqueness of children and families and the ways that practitioners respect that uniqueness. In addition, video exemplars accompany the book. To see and hear what the intervention is like can make all the difference.

A child hears an airplane, looks to the sky, then looks at Dad and back to the sky. Without words, the child has said, "Hey, Dad, look at that airplane." Another child looks at the bit of cereal that Mom holds in one hand as she holds a cracker in the other. Mom asks, "Do you want the cereal or the cracker?" The child looks at one and then the other. She takes a longer look at the cracker, up toward Mom, and back at the cracker. Mom responds, "Oh, I see you want the cracker. Here you go." These seemingly ordinary exchanges can be anything but ordinary for young children with moderate and severe disabilities and complex communication needs. Yet, these sorts of interactions are the foundation of development and learning. We can thank Lesley Olswang, Julie L. Feuerstein, and Gay Lloyd Pinder for sharing their research and expertise so that more young children and families may experience the delight of interaction, engagement, and intentional communication.

Susan R. Sandall, Ph.D.
Professor Emeritus, College of Education
University of Washington

Acknowledgments

We wish to acknowledge a number of people whose contributions were essential to this book. We recognize the significant contribution of Dr. Patricia Dowden, who was part of our team for many years at the University of Washington. Dr. Dowden's dedication to improving the lives of children with disabilities and complex communication needs and their families has been tireless. Her passion for helping these children successfully communicate motivated our team to challenge our own thinking and continually improve the Triadic Gaze Intervention (TGI) program. Four other members of our team were integral to the design of TGI and the testing of its effectiveness: Tina Watkinson, Jodi Madden, Becca Hanson, and Kathryn Greenslade. A special thank you to Tina, who not only provided skill and caring to TGI over the years but also became our sounding board through the writing of this book as we sought her wisdom about current early intervention (EI) practices. Jodi worked magic with "her families" with her practical and imaginative approach to TGI. Her insights are present throughout this book. Becca was parent-focused and is remembered with affection by the families with whom she worked. Finally, Kathryn was extraordinary in helping with so many aspects of developing TGI. We welcomed with great appreciation her particular talents with organizing, coding, and verifying our data. We also wish to thank our colleagues at the University of Kansas who collaborated on the later stages of our research and provided leadership in the investigation of the Communication Complexity Scale. A special acknowledgment and gratitude go to all the participants (children, caregivers, and practitioners) and the many University of Washington students who contributed to our three decades of research. The administration and practitioners at Children's Therapy Center of Kent, Washington deserve particular recognition for their time and belief in examining the benefits of TGI over the years. They were critical collaborators in connecting us with families and testing our protocol in practice. A special thank you goes to Melissa Behm, Liz Gildea, Tess Hoffman, and MaryBeth Winkler, as well as others at Brookes for their guidance and effort in bringing this book and ideas to publication. Finally, with full hearts, we recognize and thank our individual families for their continual support of our effort in bringing this book to completion:

- *Lesley Olswang:* To my husband, Steven, thank you for your tireless caring, endless energy, and stunning good cheer that has supported my work over the years. Your insights, enthusiasm, and love have contributed to this book in more ways than you will ever know. And to my boys, Benjamin and Harrison, and their families, thank you for all the ways you have enabled my efforts to understand communication development and disorders, most importantly, by bringing joy and balance to my life. Finally, to my former students and colleagues, thank you for the many meaningful conversations that have shaped my thinking.

- *Julie L. Feuerstein:* To my husband, Ross, who believed in this book and in me, and who over the past year and through a pandemic made certain that I had the time and space to devote to this work. And to my children, Mara and Ayla, who constantly remind me of the beautiful and magical power of engagement, connection, and communication.

- *Gay Lloyd Pinder:* To my partner, Jean, who patiently shared our time and my focus during this productive effort to publish the knowledge gained during these 30-plus years of work together.

To all the children and families who helped shape this book

SECTION I

Understanding Early Communication Development and Triadic Gaze Intervention

CHAPTER 1

The Child–Adult Dance and the Gift of Engagement and Communication

The first year of life is instinctively dominated by nurturing moments between babies and **families**, filled with holding, feeding, and socializing. Imagine the beautiful dance that takes place between adult and child as they become finely tuned partners learning to engage and communicate with each other. Children grow and thrive in the context of close and dependable relationships that provide a safe and predictable environment and encourage exploration (National Research Council & Institute of Medicine, 2000). Research has overwhelmingly demonstrated the importance of these first relationships to build a strong foundation for children's future social-emotional, language, and cognitive learning (Bakeman & Brown, 1980; Brazelton, 1982, 1988; Bruner, 1983; Kelly et al., 2008). The fundamental ingredient for these early moments is the reciprocal interaction (i.e., turn taking) that takes place between adult and child.

As the adult and child get to know each other, they become exquisite dance partners interacting throughout the day in all types of activities and situations. Arnold Sameroff and colleagues have described this dynamic back-and-forth behavior between child and adult in their well-accepted Transactional Model (Fiese & Sameroff, 1989; Sameroff, 1987; Sameroff & Fiese, 1990). The connection established between the adult and child, as shown in the photo in Figure 1.1, sets the stage and provides the context for all kinds of future learning. Regardless of the child's age, or the circumstances, these types of interactions capture the gift of engagement.

This chapter briefly describes the natural emergence of engagement and the development of early communication during the first year of life. The way in which child–adult interactions form the context for early learning is explained, including how the nature of these interactions supports not only communication but also learning across developmental domains. The chapter then describes in detail children's early communication, defining specific, conventional preverbal behaviors (i.e., **gaze,** gestures, vocalizations) that become intentional forms of communication. So much happens before children talk; this chapter ends with a discussion of how preverbal communication emerges and leads to first words and word combinations.

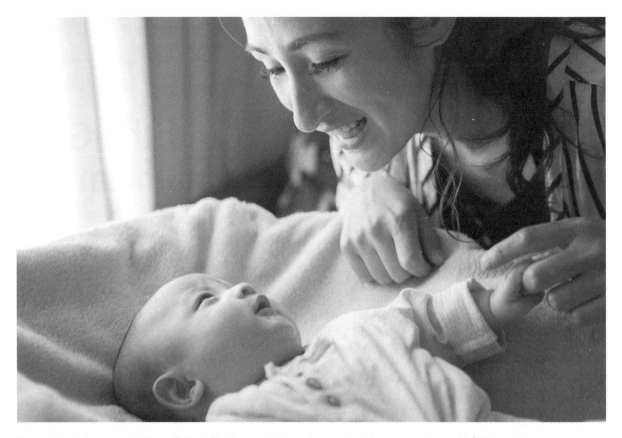

Figure 1.1.   Early communication as illustrated by the eye contact and engagement between mother and infant.

EARLY ENGAGEMENT: THE CONTEXT FOR LEARNING

The context for early engagement, learning to communicate, and in fact, all future learning, is naturally present from birth. The caregiver holds the infant, and the stage is set. Engagement begins with the infant's first cries and whimpers; they serve to immediately engage the adult. These early **reflexive behaviors** effectively grab the adult and set up the context for interaction. As the days and weeks go by, these critically important exchanges continue. Gradually the adult begins to give meaning to the infant's behaviors of crying, cooing, gazing, and early smiling, responding to them consistently and, in turn, setting up dependable back-and-forth routines that the baby can trust (Adamson & Dimitrova, 2014).

These interactive routines will occur throughout all kinds of activities, including feeding, bath time, and social play, which then serve as natural opportunities for supporting engagement and shared attention between adult and child (Bruner, 1999; Dunst et al., 2000). Routines start simply via mutual exchange of gaze between the adult and infant as the infant is held. The adult gradually adds more to the interaction by starting to socially play with the infant, for example, by making sounds, tickling, and kissing. The adult eventually will introduce objects (e.g., food items, toys) during activities. Once this happens, the interaction between adult and child becomes more complicated and sophisticated, as the child has the opportunity to coordinate their attention to both adult and object (Adamson et al., 2014).

During these early interactions, the adult is structuring the environment to encourage engagement and communication, and also is paying attention and responding to the child's efforts to connect. These profound interactions occur long before spoken language emerges; yet, they are the very interactions that support language development. During these interactive contexts, the child is learning to pay attention to people, objects, and relationships between them. They are also learning to listen and map the adult words onto these objects and actions. In fact, research has clearly shown that early engagement of these kinds, and specifically those involving coordinated joint attention among child, adult, and objects, is associated with later social-emotional, cognitive, and language development. (See Adamson & Dimitrova, 2014, and Mundy & Newell, 2007, for thorough reviews of this research.)

Engaged interactions between adult and child are critical for learning. The adult brings the necessary structure, providing opportunities for engagement but also skills for recognizing the child's signals of attention and interpreting the child's wants and needs. Of course, the adult needs a partner; research has shown the adult will only continue to engage if the child is an active participant in the exchange (Murray & Trevarthen, 1986). Let's turn now to examining more closely what the child brings to this learning environment and how these behaviors rope in the adult to create a magnificent turn-taking dance between child and adult, which shapes development.

CHILD BEHAVIORS AND THE EMERGENCE OF INTENTIONAL COMMUNICATION

Early communication behaviors produced by infants and toddlers begin long before first words. These **preverbal communication behaviors** typically include gaze, gestures, and vocalizations and emerge along a **communication continuum** in three phases: **preintentional**, **intentional**, and **symbolic communication** (e.g., Bates et al., 1975; Locke, 1993; Thomasello, 1999). Brady and colleagues (Brady et al., 2012; Salley et al., 2019) delineated this continuum of behaviors in the Communication Complexity Scale (CCS; 2012). The CCS was designed to observe and assess specific **prelinguistic forms** of communication in children and adults who are nonverbal. With this purpose, the CCS defines a sequence of conventionally recognizable preverbal behaviors (i.e., gaze, gestures, and vocalizations) that have been documented as preceding symbolic language (i.e., first words, signs, or symbols; word, sign, and/or symbol combinations).

Reminder: A lot happens before first words!

Gaze, because of its powerful and definitive interactive signal, serves as the anchor behavior in the continuum, moving from single focus, to dual focus, to triadic focus. As will be described, gaze can be accompanied by gestures and vocalizations to further clarify the engagement and message. As children develop, frequency and complexity of these behaviors increase (Salley et al., 2019). Figure 1.2 illustrates the continuum of preverbal behaviors, which will serve to guide the following description of early communication, from preintentional, to intentional, to symbolic.

Preintentional Communication: Single Focus

An infant's very first behaviors are **reflexive behaviors** and include eye gaze, body orientation and movements, and bodily noises that suggest engaged and disengaged infant states (Kelly et al., 2008). During the first 3 months of life, the engaged behaviors include, for

Preintentional

Single focus: looking and sustaining gaze to a person OR an object
- Gaze alone
- Gaze + gestures OR vocalizations
- Gaze + gestures AND vocalizations

Dual focus: looking from an object to a person OR a person to an object
- Gaze alone
- Gaze + gestures OR vocalizations
- Gaze + gestures AND vocalizations

Triadic focus: looking back and forth between an object and a person (person-object-person OR object-person-object)
- Gaze alone
- Gaze + gestures OR vocalizations
- Gaze + gestures AND vocalizations

Intentional

Figure 1.2.   Preverbal communication behaviors: Foundation for first words. (Adapted from Brady et al., 2012.) Republished with permission of American Speech-Language-Hearing Association, from *Development of the Communication Complexity Scale*, Brady, N., Fleming, K., Thiemann-Bourke, K, Olswang, L., Dowden, P., & Saunders, M., *21*(1), 2012; permission conveyed through Copyright Clearance Center, Inc.

example, having eyes open, looking intently, feeding, or making sounds of contentment. Disengaged behaviors, in contrast, might include grimacing, squealing, crying, or turning away. Lots of guessing occurs during these early months as parents try to determine their children's wants and needs. Over time, the infant becomes more organized in response to the environment, and gross movements become increasingly more precise as motor control develops.

As children naturally develop, their behaviors become more distinct and recognizable. As such they are more purposeful. Emerging first is a clear **single focus** orientation and gaze to an adult and then gradually to objects. This can be observed as early as age 4 months as children develop increased head control. The child will begin to move from being oriented to an adult, to glancing at the adult, to sustaining a gaze with the adult. Think about how a child will begin staring at the adult's face. This single focus, which is an early form of social joint attention between child and adult, gradually begins to include objects (e.g., bottle, rattle): quickly or passively glancing at objects and eventually maintaining an active look toward them. By around 5 months of age, a child's trunk control allows for more purposeful and regulated gazing, even accompanied by gestures (e.g., leaning, reaching) and vocalizations (e.g., vowel sounds, consonant-like sounds). However, the child at this stage does *not* link the adult to the object. Consider how a child might begin paying attention to the pet dog or staring at the mobile above their crib. The child might make sounds and try to reach, but the focus is clearly on only the object or the adult, one at a time. These are certainly **purposeful behaviors**, but they do not yet indicate intentional communication.

Preintentional Communication: Dual Focus

Single focus gradually moves to the child purposefully following the adult's gaze to other people or objects. This emerging expression of joint attention is always exciting as it appears the child is noticing more about their world. The child will increasingly and more definitively reach, at first to the adult and then to others, including objects. Think about a child reaching for the bottle during feeding or splashing the water during bath time. This has been termed **dual focus**. Note how the gaze becomes more complex as shown in Figure 1.2. Gaze and gestures will increasingly be accompanied by vocalizations, which too are becoming more complex (e.g., consonant–vowel combinations).

Between 8 and 10 months, children's production of these behaviors noticeably increases in frequency and complexity, which in turn expands their social, joint attention moments with others. These behaviors, although becoming more and more frequent and purposeful, are not necessarily meant to intentionally communicate with others; yet, they serve to make interactions more readable and gratifying. Consider a child gazing at a mobile and trying to reach for it while having their diaper changed. The parent might regard this as a comment on the mobile or a request for it, but there is really no evidence for intentional communication on the child's part. Yet, the adult will typically acknowledge these behaviors with an attentive remark. As described previously, these are the early forms that build a child's ability to engage with others. As the child increases their behavioral repertoire, the adult will find these potentially communicative behaviors easier to recognize and interpret.

Families will respond more frequently to discrete, clear behaviors and less frequently to the more global, hard-to-read ones, thereby shaping the infant's more refined communicative attempts. For example, families will more readily interpret a child's looking at a bottle and vocalizing "uh uh uh" while reaching toward it as a request for wanting a drink than they will interpret a child's quickly looking at the bottle while arching their back and fussing as a request. As the child gains and uses more conventional and readable behaviors (more intent gazes, more definitive gestures, and more varied vocalizations), the adult will be more consistent in responding. Through this back-and-forth, the child begins to learn that these early behaviors cause the adult to do something. This is the magical turn-taking dance between adult and child that provides the structure of language learning. Meanwhile, the child is also becoming increasingly interested in objects in the environment and bringing them into the interaction.

During this period of development, children are more purposely acting on their environment (people and objects) but are not yet linking the two as is necessary in intentional communication. Not until the child begins to knowingly direct their behaviors to another person, for the purpose of influencing that person, is the child said to be communicating with intentionality (Bakeman & Adamson, 1984; Bates et al., 1975; Locke, 1993; Thomasello, 1999). What does intentional communication look like?

Intentional Communication: Triadic Focus

Some time around 9–10 months of age, a dramatic milestone can be observed; the child begins shifting their gaze back and forth between an adult and an object or event of interest; this is called **triadic focus**, as indicated in Figure 1.2. The significance of triadic gaze, defined by a clear three-point gaze shift, or back-and-forth looking (often accompanied by gestures and vocalizations), between an adult and an object or event of interest, is the behavioral indication that the child is linking the adult to an action or object for the purpose of getting the adult to act in some way. This has been described as **intentional communication** prior to first words (Bakeman & Adamson, 1984; Bates et al., 1975; Locke, 1993; Trevarthen & Hubley, 1978).

As a child is moving from dual to triadic focus, they are also experiencing many opportunities to explore and act on objects, gaining knowledge about making things happen, and learning about their power to cause an effect on the world (i.e., means–ends relationships). This object experience coincides with the exposure the child is having to adults responding consistently to the child's preintentional communication attempts. The coming together of the child's knowledge of objects and adults, and relationships between them, as well as the adults' responsiveness to early behaviors, appears to facilitate the emergence of intentional communication (Bakeman & Adamson, 1984; Bates et al., 1975; Locke, 1993; Trevarthen & Hubley, 1978).

Salley and colleagues (2019) observed that the frequency, complexity, and readability of children's behaviors continue to increase through 12 months of age, making communication a more active and reciprocal part of interactions between children and adults. Families become better at recognizing children's behaviors and interpreting their intentions. The exchange reflects a dialogue between children and others, even before first words are spoken. The triadic gaze milestone not only marks intentionality, but it has also been associated with significant neurological change and has been shown to be predictive of later language development (Beuker et al., 2013; McCathren & Warren, 1996; Mundy & Newell, 2007; Mundy et al., 1990). **Triadic Gaze Intervention (TGI)** is named to acknowledge the significance of this early prelinguistic milestone and the importance of an intervention designed to facilitate its accomplishment.

A video montage of four children is provided in **Video 1.1, Typical Development,** to illustrate babies' typical development of preverbal communication behaviors. (This video, along with other videos illustrating communication behaviors and TGI components, is available on the Brookes Download Hub with the downloadable resources for this book. See "About the Video Clips and Downloads" at the front of the book for details about how to access this content.)

The children in Video 1.1 produce conventional nonverbal behaviors of gaze, gestures, and vocalizations as they emerge during the first 12 months of life. As you watch these children interact with an adult (or in one case, the baby's older sibling), note how they use their behaviors to engage and communicate. The video clips are arranged in order of sophistication, illustrating the continuum of behaviors listed in Figure 1.2, moving from single focus, to dual focus, and ultimately to triadic focus. The sequence of videos also illustrates emerging postural stability that supports the children's developing communication behaviors.

The first two children in the montage primarily use single focus toward an object to communicate. The first child is given a choice between a stuffed animal and a rattle. Note how he looks between the objects and uses single gaze alone to make a choice. The second child is offered a ball for play. She also uses single focus but adds a lean and reach to communicate. The next two children are developmentally further along the communication continuum. The third child in the montage is offered a choice between a ball and a ducky. Note her quick back-and-forth looking between objects and her sister as she reaches toward the ducky. Though her behaviors are quick, they appear more purposeful. The fourth and final child in the video montage demonstrates the most sophisticated communication behaviors by producing a clear triadic gaze when choosing between a stuffed animal and a tambourine. Note how the child scans the objects and includes the adult, finally, looking between the stuffed animal and Mom while reaching and vocalizing. The montage of the four children illustrates how preverbal behaviors, and, therefore, the communicative attempts, become clearer and clearer from the first video clip to the last. With the clarity, the communication partner has an easier and easier time interpreting the child's intention. This video montage is meant to illustrate typical development and serve as a reference for understanding preverbal communication and all that happens before first words.

Symbolic Communication: Emergence of Word Approximations and First Words

As children reach their first birthday, their behaviors become even more discrete and clear, including vocalizations that move from simple consonant–vowel productions to more complex sound combinations. Eventually these sound combinations become forms that resemble word approximations and, from here, first words. So, too, do gestures increase in variety and clarity, moving from leaning and reaching, to showing, giving, and pointing. These vocal and gestural behaviors that accompany triadic gaze contribute to an explosion of communicative activity. Children's efforts to communicate grow exponentially, as do the clarity and meaning of their intentions. Between 15 and 18 months, families attribute the production of many words to their children, along with a variety of **communicative intentions**. The turn taking in communication becomes almost second nature between children and adults: Asking and answering becomes part of most, if not all, routines. Preverbal development of gaze, gestures, and vocalizations is rich and predictable in form, moving from hard to read and interpret, to clear signals of intentional communication.

Communicative Intentions

Coggins and Carpenter (1981) and Carpenter and colleagues (1983) identified a variety of intentions that children express prior to first words, moving from simple preverbal behaviors to more complex ones. Coggins and Carpenter (1981) demonstrated that children use these early behaviors for protesting, requesting (objects, actions, and information), commenting (on actions and objects), acknowledging, and answering. In a small longitudinal study of mothers interacting with their children between the ages of 8 and 16 months, Carpenter and colleagues (1983) found that preverbal forms of protesting, requesting, and commenting were observed most frequently. This work demonstrates that gaze, gestures, and vocalizations can be reliably observed and interpreted as expressing a variety of communicative intents. Table 1.1 provides examples of these early communicative intentions and illustrates why and how preverbal children communicate prior to first words. The literature clearly supports the developmental progression of preverbal behaviors and the way children use these behaviors to communicate. This development is crucial as a foundation for launching first words, signs, and/or augmentative and alternative communication symbols.

The emergence of the child's behaviors occurs during the natural turn-taking interactions between child and caregiver as described previously. It is the back and forth, give and take of engaged, reciprocal interactions in the context of daily activities around social events and object play that provide the foundation for learning language. Important to remember is that the success of the interaction is the give and take between adult and child. Both the adult and child are active participants in the interaction and meaningfully contribute to maintaining a successful connection (Murray & Trevarthen, 1986). The clarity of the child's behaviors has been found to be extremely important for the parent to be

Table 1.1. Examples of preverbal communicative intentions

Common communicative intentions	Example of preverbal behaviors	Apparent meaning
Protesting	Mother offers her child a bottle. Child looks away, pushes bottle away, and fusses.	"I don't want that."
Requesting		
Actions	Child and mother are playing peekaboo. Mother is covering and uncovering her eyes. Mother stops. Child looks at her mom, gets fidgety, squeals, and vocalizes "uh uh uh."	"I want more peekaboo game."
Objects	Child looks at and points to a book on a shelf, looks at his mother, looks back to the book, and vocalizes "da" persistently until mother gives the book to the child.	"Give me that book."
Commenting		
On actions	Child looks at brother doing somersaults on the grass. Child smiles, squeals, and waves her arms each time her brother tumbles.	"Look at that!"
On objects	Dog comes and sits beside the child. Child looks at the dog, reaches toward the dog, looks at mother and then back to the dog, and vocalizes "da."	"Dog."
Answering	Mother asks her child if she wants to swing. Child looks at mother and vocalizes "ah ah."	"Yes, I want to swing."

Sources: Coggins & Carpenter, 1981; Carpenter et al., 1983.

able to fulfill their role in providing feedback to the child (Brazelton, 1982; Bruner, 1982). For some children with disabilities, behaviors are limited and, in turn, interactions with families disrupted. Children with motor, social, or cognitive challenges may have particular difficulty producing conventional early preverbal behaviors, resulting in **caregivers** being challenged in deciphering and interpreting what their children want and need. When this happens, the rhythm and synchrony between adult and child during interactions can be interrupted. In the case of prolonged disturbance of reciprocal interactions, as might occur with children who have moderate to severe disabilities, the parents may become less responsive to the children's attempts. Finally, in addition to the early disruption of the social-communicative interaction, the child's experiences with objects may also be affected. The result ultimately may put a child's development in jeopardy.

CONCLUSION

A lot happens in communication development prior to first words. The beautiful dance that occurs between adults and children as they interact during the first 12 months of life reflects children's gradual development of behaviors (e.g., gaze, gestures, vocalizations) that caregivers recognize and interpret as early forms of communication. The dance reflects ongoing turn taking, with caregivers better able to read their children's behaviors and children increasingly producing more frequent and complex combinations of behaviors. Both become skilled at reading and responding to each other. For some children with disabilities, behaviors may be challenging to produce and, in turn, will interfere with their ability to engage and communicate with others. Triadic Gaze Intervention, as described in this book, is designed to address breakdowns in the child–adult dance and provide a strategy for bringing the partners back into synchrony. We turn now to a discussion of children with disabilities, their possible challenges in engaging and communicating, and available approaches to support these children and their families.

CHAPTER **2**

When the Dance Is Interrupted

Young Children With Disabilities and Intervention

The previous chapter reviewed the emergence of intentional communication in children developing typically, in the context of shared connections with their caregivers. The synchronous back-and-forth interactions between children and their caregivers powerfully build engagement and preverbal communication behaviors that culminate in first words. This chapter discusses how disabilities can have an impact on development in young children who have complex communication needs, which, in turn, may alter the typical interactions they have with their caregivers. The chapter continues with a discussion of early intervention that focuses on engagement and communication, laying the groundwork for the creation of TGI and the research program that has investigated its efficacy.

YOUNG CHILDREN WITH DISABILITIES

Young children with moderate to severe disabilities (e.g., cerebral palsy, congenital conditions, genetic syndromes, autism spectrum disorder, Down syndrome) constitute a diverse group who can be affected by impairments across sensory, motor, cognitive, and social-emotional domains. Some children may have sensory or perceptual impairments, including hearing and vision deficits, or high/low sensitivity to auditory, visual, and/or tactile stimulation. Many also may exhibit a range of motor impairments, including hypotonic to hypertonic muscle tone. Some require supportive positioning to establish head, neck, and/or trunk control, whereas others may exhibit extremely subtle motor problems. Cognitive delays may also challenge some children because of neurological involvement and limited ability to explore the environment (e.g., knowledge of objects, object relations such as means–end). Furthermore, the cognitive abilities of these children are difficult to assess. As a result, the true level of cognitive function may be unknown for years. Finally, these children may demonstrate social-emotional problems. These challenges may understandably accompany sensory, motor, and cognitive deficits. Complicating all of these developmental problems, some children can experience unstable health, with accompanying seizure disorders and feeding difficulties threatening survival. Whether mild, moderate, or severe, the array of problems can result in significant day-to-day performance variability that impairs interactions and eventual communication development (Dowden & Cook, 2012).

Complex Communication Needs

A term that has proven valuable in describing this population of children with diverse profiles is **individuals with complex communication needs** (CCN) (Beukelman & Light, 2020; Beukelman & Mirenda, 2005, 2013; Iacono, 2014). CCN describes challenges that interfere with connecting with others and the possibility of not using speech as a primary means of communication (Iacono, 2014). As should be apparent, the impairments that these children exhibit may limit their production of gestures, gaze, vocalizations, and even facial expressions, which provide the foundation for engaging with others (Sigafoos & Mirenda, 2002).

Effects on Children's Communicative Behaviors

When these foundational communicative behaviors are unclear or absent, children with CCN may begin to produce idiosyncratic behaviors in an attempt to engage caregivers (Sigafoos & Mirenda, 2002). Motor limitations may certainly affect the production of clear gestures and vocalizations, but so might sensory and cognitive challenges. Sometimes, young children with moderate to severe disabilities may persist in the production of less conventional early behaviors that prove to be counterproductive (e.g., arching the back, full body extension, screaming) (Pinder & Olswang, 1995; Pinder et al., 1993). Iacono and colleagues (1998) also have documented the use of unconventional behaviors in these children, for example, "stereotypic behaviors" and repetitions of motor behaviors. Other children may start to use conventional orientation and gaze behaviors; however, because their productions may be compromised due to poor motor control or limitations in production of accompanying gestures and vocalizations, caregivers may not readily recognize and respond to these behaviors. These children may then revert to less sophisticated or unconventional forms. Important to note is that some children's disabilities may be so extensive that they limit the production of conventional behaviors. In these cases, their attempts and approximations need to be recognized and respected. This will require close scrutiny to determine if children are producing subtle behaviors (e.g., a single finger movement, slight full body alerting) that potentially could be communicative.

Effects on Reciprocal Communicative Interactions

All of these developmental limitations pose challenges to engagement and communication with others. Unclear, ambiguous, or absent behaviors on the part of the child will very likely be difficult for caregivers to recognize and interpret. In these cases, the back-and-forth dance between adult and child can be interrupted. If this happens, the children's deficits will likely have a negative effect on their ability to participate fully in natural reciprocal interactions, which in turn may result in their missing out on important teaching and learning opportunities that occur with caregivers (Halle et al., 2004; Iacono et al., 1998; Paparella & Kasari, 2004). As time goes by, the communicative interactions between child and adult may become more challenging, resulting in increasing frustration for both and possibly fewer constructive play and social interaction opportunities. At a very basic level, the children and their caregivers will miss crucial opportunities for the all-important turn taking that drives development.

To illustrate, consider a child who produces a quick lean or a fleeting, passive glance to a piece of banana when given a choice between two snack items, banana and cereal. The caregiver may not notice this behavior or recognize it as the child showing their preference. The difficulty the adult experiences in recognizing the child's signal, and the possibility of misinterpretation, might lead to the child fussing or worse. This interaction might lead to extinguishing the lean-and-look behavior and even reinforce the disruptive behavior. Another child might be so engrossed in an activity (e.g., a windup toy that produces sounds and lights) that when it stops, the child's excitement about the toy triggers a full-body extension with vocalizations. In this case, the caregiver might understand that the child wants more, but by recognizing and acknowledging this behavior, the caregiver will be inadvertently reinforcing it. This course of interaction, if repeated, might serve to interfere with more conventional forms of requesting.

Families need and want to understand and appreciate their children's engagement and communicative attempts. The challenge for the adult is recognizing these attempts, which may be unconventional or subtle, and responding, thus facilitating a reciprocal interaction. On top of these profound social-communicative challenges, these children very often have limited experiences with important play activities of exploring and manipulating objects, either singularly or in relationship with other objects. Interruptions in opportunities to learn about objects in the context of interacting (playing) with adults can significantly limit the child's recognition that they can purposely direct another person to act by producing particular behaviors (i.e., learn to intentionally communicate). These challenges to children and their families should be addressed through early support services offered by professionals. Because engagement and communication are foundational to cognitive, social-emotional, and language development, **practitioners** are advised to pay close attention to child and family needs in this area. Services might directly focus on engagement and communication skills and abilities or make these a part of other goals. Most importantly, early preverbal engagement and communication should not be neglected.

OVERVIEW OF EFFECTIVE INTERVENTIONS

The need to address engagement and communication in early intervention for children with developmental disabilities has clearly been supported in the literature (Brady & Warren, 2003; Hebbeler et al., 2007; Kasari et al., 2001; Kelly et al., 2008; Trevarthen & Aitken, 2001; Woods & Wetherby, 2003; Yoder & Warren, 1993). One particular intervention, *Promoting First Relationships* (Kelly et al., 2008), is designed to support caregivers in building confidence and knowledge in interacting with their at-risk young children to facilitate positive child developmental outcomes. This intervention is built on attachment principles that nurture social-emotional development during natural adult–child interactions. It has primarily focused on toddlers and caregivers in child welfare and in foster care, and children referred to Child Protective Services, with a curriculum for building sensitive, nurturing relationships. (See more about the intervention at the Promoting First Relationships web site at https://pfrprogram.org/research/nih-funded-randomized-trials/.)

Several valuable, popular interventions have been established over the years to facilitate communication and language acquisition through caregiver training, including *It Takes Two to Talk (The Hanen Program)* (Girolametto, 1988; Tannock et al., 1992), *Responsivity Education/Prelinguistic Milieu Teaching (RE/PMT)* (Warren et al., 2006), and *Enhanced Milieu Teaching (EMT)* (Kaiser & Roberts, 2013; Windsor et al., 2019). These interventions emphasize the importance of caregiver-implemented strategies during routine activities throughout the day to enhance their young children's early communication and language.

Two other early intervention programs that support young children and families in encouraging development through natural interactions are the *Social Communication Emotional Regulation Transactional Support Model (SCERTS®)* (Prizant et al., 2006) and the *Joint Attention,*

Symbolic Play, Engagement & Regulation (JASPER) (Kasari et al., 2001; Paparella & Kasari, 2004). These approaches are intended for children with autism spectrum disorder and their families and reflect many of the theories and principles related to early engagement.

All of the interventions noted here have strong conceptual and empirical foundations. They recognize the power of reciprocal interactions and teaching and learning within naturally occurring daily activities. They also share their emphasis on selecting developmentally appropriate goals and teaching strategies. In these ways, the interventions overlap with each other and the intervention being described in this book. However, each is unique and arguably offers something different for practitioners, families, and children. Most apparent is that they each differ in their targeted primary population of children with disabilities and CCN, and rather more subtly in their treatment focus and desired outcomes.

TRIADIC GAZE INTERVENTION

Given so many useful interventions, what would prompt the need for another one? The intervention described in this publication, TGI, was designed to fill a gap in treatment for very young children with moderate to severe disabilities and their families as they encounter challenges in engaging and communicating with each other during their first years of life. TGI is a strategy for focusing on early engagement and communication by helping families recognize their children's communication attempts and increase their children's repertoire of conventional communication behaviors that will, in turn, encourage more successful interactions. TGI recognizes the importance of early engagement and communication and prioritizes it in services to children with CCN and their families. Since the early 1990s, a research team at the University of Washington, Department of Speech and Hearing Sciences, has been developing and refining an intervention designed specifically for very young children (10–24 months) with moderate to severe disabilities and CCN who experience challenges when sending clear signals to engage with caregivers. Because of the children's primary sensory and motor problems, they exhibit noticeable difficulties with the all-important foundational opportunities to engage with their families in activities of daily living, including play with objects.

TGI was created to address two unique and critical objectives for these children and their families: 1) increase children's production of more conventional preverbal behaviors (gaze, gestures, vocalizations), which reflect engagement, and build toward triadic gaze as a clear signal of intentional communication; and 2) help families provide

> **TGI**
> Recognizes and prioritizes engagement and communication in early support services for children with disabilities and their families.
>
> TGI was created to meet two objectives:
>
> 1. Increase children's productions of more conventional preverbal behaviors (gaze, gestures, and vocalizations) which reflect engagement and build toward triadic gaze as a clear signal of intentional communication.
> 2. Help families provide deliberate opportunities for engagement; recognize and reinforce their children's communicative attempts; and when possible, encourage more sophisticated, intentional communication behaviors.

deliberate opportunities for engagement; recognize and reinforce their children's communicative attempts; and when possible, encourage more sophisticated, intentional communication behaviors. TGI was built on strong theoretical constructs, principles, and research related to the Transactional Model, joint attention, and communication development as described in Chapter 1. In its own right, the TGI strategy has been shown to be an effective way to facilitate engaged interactions and shape children's clear and conventional signals that lead to intentional communication as indicated by triadic gaze, and even encourage play with objects. TGI capitalizes on recognizing often overlooked, potentially communicative behaviors and building supportive communicative contexts to enable children with compromised motor abilities and other developmental impairments to successfully interact with people and objects in their environment. TGI prioritizes early engagement and communication in early support services to families. It targets engagement by structuring the natural environment to facilitate communicative opportunities and recognizing children's preverbal attempts to interact, and by shaping those behaviors into recognizable, productive communication signals. TGI recognizes intentional communication as foundational for later learning!

EVIDENCE SUPPORTING TGI

The evidence supporting TGI and its objectives has accumulated over almost three decades. During this time period, the actual treatment protocol associated with TGI became more specific, but the overall conceptual strategy remained the same. Initial studies explored the feasibility of an early form of the protocol designed to teach triadic gaze. These studies were followed by a larger randomized controlled study using a refined, delineated protocol designated **PoWRRS-Connect** as an acronym for its six essential elements: **provide opportunity**, **wait**, **recognize** the child's behavior, **respond**, **shape**, and **connect.** This randomized controlled study involved more practitioners and children with diverse characteristics. Finally, implementation studies were completed to examine training with EI practitioners, examining their fidelity in the administration of the PoWRRS-Connect protocol used to implement TGI and their perceptions of the intervention in practice. Table 2.1 summarizes the evolving research program and resulting evidence that was completed across three decades.

Table 2.1. Summary of three decades of research supporting Triadic Gaze Intervention (TGI)

Evidence supporting TGI

Feasibility studies
- Demonstrated the success of TGI treatment in increasing intentional preverbal communication behaviors during structured toy play activities with a speech-language pathologist
- Demonstrated the success of TGI treatment in increasing intentional preverbal communication behaviors during toy play and snack activities with caregivers
- Demonstrated TGI treatment not only increased communication behaviors but also children's interest and sophistication in playing with toys or objects

Case-controlled study
- Demonstrated the success of TGI, implemented through the PoWRRS-Connect treatment protocol, by three different speech-language pathologists, for increasing the production of triadic gaze as an intentional communication behavior with a large number of children with varied degrees of disabilities
- Documented the validity of dynamic assessment procedures for determining which preverbal communication behaviors to target for treatment using TGI

Implementation studies
- Demonstrated the fidelity of practitioners from a variety of birth-to-three services in implementing the PoWRRS-Connect protocol
- Demonstrated the value of the structure provided by TGI for addressing children's and families' needs during everyday routines
- Demonstrated that aspects of the PoWRRS-Connect protocol could be taught to EI practitioners online

Feasibility Studies

Several single subject studies explored the benefits of treatment to teach early communication behaviors for children diagnosed specifically with cerebral palsy (Pinder, Olswang, & Coggins, 1993; Pinder & Olswang, 1995). These early empirical studies demonstrated the success of the treatment in structured play contexts with a speech-language pathologist. They also demonstrated that the communicative behaviors were most easily elicited during activities that required the child to request an object or action. The success of TGI treatment when administered by parents during play and snack activities was also examined and demonstrated that the treatment increased the children's production of dual and triadic gaze behaviors (Olswang et al., 2006). This research also demonstrated aspects of the treatment that were most successfully learned by parents. Finally, the research demonstrated that treatment not only increased production of triadic gaze but also increased the children's interest and sophistication in manipulating objects or toys during play activities (Olswang & Pinder, 1995).

Case-Controlled Study

The efficacy of the treatment was further explored in a randomized controlled study, which investigated the production of triadic gaze by children enrolled in TGI versus children enrolled in standard care (Olswang et al., 2014). Children in the TGI group received services via speech-language pathologists implementing the PoWRRS-Connect protocol in the natural environment. Children in the standard care group received services through birth-to-three centers in either center or natural environments. This between-group study demonstrated the promise of the TGI strategy utilizing the PoWRRS-Connect protocol for teaching children with diverse clinical characteristics to use triadic gaze with or without gestures and vocalizations as a preverbal intentional signal of communication (Olswang et al., 2014). Another study documented the validity of the dynamic assessment portion of TGI for determining which preverbal communicative behaviors to target for individual children (Olswang et al., 2013). This study demonstrated that the assessment procedures (an abbreviated form of PoWRRS-Connect) were successful in determining not only which behaviors to treat but also which children were most likely to benefit from the treatment.

Implementation Studies

The documented success of TGI and the PoWRRS-Connect protocol in these studies was followed by a series of studies exploring implementation in practice. This research involved practitioners representing speech-language pathology, occupational therapy, and physical therapy. The research explored the practitioners' fidelity in delivering the PoWRRS-Connect protocol and practitioners' views on adopting TGI in their clinical routines (Feuerstein et al., 2017, 2018). The first study demonstrated practitioners' abilities to accurately administer the PoWRRS-Connect protocol. The second study documented practitioners' opinions about the TGI strategy. They described TGI as beneficial for giving them focus in addressing children's and families' needs, offering structure to their service delivery, and appreciating the importance of gaze as a preverbal form of communication (Feuerstein et al., 2018). One practitioner commented,

> I just started working with this little guy, and I feel like it gives me such a nice framework to work with him—what are the next steps, what are we doing right now, what are those really concrete strategies we can pass along to parents. . . it's really been helpful. (Feuerstein et al., 2018, p. 652)

Finally, a training study was conducted to investigate whether aspects of the PoWRRS-Connect protocol could be taught to practitioners online (Feuerstein & Olswang, 2020). This study demonstrated the relative merits of three different online training conditions for learning to recognize preverbal communication behaviors. Furthermore, the study explored practitioners' perceptions and appeal of the different online learning conditions. (See Appendix A for details regarding the full TGI research program and accumulated evidence.)

Taken together, this research program has documented the benefits of TGI. The supportive evidence and the positive reception by practitioners and parents motivated the publication of this intervention in the current book. It fills an important niche in early support services by providing specific guidance to help children with moderate to severe disabilities and CCN and their families build positive, reciprocal interactions. TGI was designed for those children and their families who are struggling to connect. Families of young children with moderate to severe disabilities are often at a loss during the first year of life for ways to help their children and to improve their ability to manage daily routines with them. TGI offers these families, and the practitioners guiding these families, a valuable support not only for making day-to-day activities go more smoothly but also for building a strong foundation for their children's future learning.

CONCLUSION

Children with moderate to severe disabilities and their families face numerous challenges early in life. A significant one is the disruption in interactions and the ability to successfully engage with others. This chapter has highlighted the nature of disabilities and the way they can interrupt the important synchronous connections between children and others. Early support services logically must address the challenges to successful engagement and communication that facilitate development. This aspect of development is often overlooked until children are older; this is a mistake. TGI prioritizes engagement and preverbal communication in early support services. It has been introduced as an important strategy to employ when meeting the needs of children with disabilities and families. We turn now to a broad discussion of early intervention, exploring the mandates that have driven service delivery over the years, how TGI evolved in this context, and how its current structure can be valuable for practitioners and families today.

CHAPTER **3**

How Triadic Gaze Intervention Evolved in the Context of Early Intervention

The TGI journey reflects the evolution of early intervention (EI) service delivery in the United States from the late 1980s to the present. Across these years, EI for children ages birth to three, and the legislation supporting EI service delivery, underwent marked adjustments. From its inception, TGI focused on early engagement and preverbal communication between children with disabilities and their families, but the context for TGI implementation changed in regard to service delivery. As EI services to children and families changed, TGI had to be adapted to meet current standards. This chapter begins with a brief overview of these national and state-wide adjustments to provide a context for TGI in EI. This will cover the U.S. federal mandates and how they are interpreted across the country. The chapter ends with a description of TGI, how it evolved over the years, how it meets current EI mandates, and suggestions for implementation.

EARLY INTERVENTION SERVICE DELIVERY EVOLVES IN THE UNITED STATES

Since the late 1980s, several changes in EI, particularly in legislation and service delivery, have affected the role of service providers and how they work with children and families, thus changing the context in which TGI is delivered. The major changes include the following:

- Part C legislation, which shifted the location of service delivery from the clinic to natural environments

- An increased focus on practitioners allying with families, influenced by the work of T. Berry Brazelton

- Emergence of a service delivery model that typically involves a transdisciplinary team with a **primary service provider** (PSP)

- Emphasis on **routines-based intervention**

The first part of this chapter discusses these changes and how they have accumulated to result in the current form of EI.

Part C Legislation and a Shift to Natural Environments

Service in the late 1980s and early 1990s was primarily conducted by a variety of professionals in clinics that served the birth-to-three population. Those practitioners typically included speech-language pathologists (SLPs), physical therapists (PTs), occupational therapists (OTs), and early educators, who were assigned to children based on their primary therapeutic and developmental needs. In 1997, the passage of the Individuals with Disabilities Education Act (IDEA) Amendments of 1997 (PL 105-17) mandated that Part C services for infants and toddlers be conducted in the least restrictive, natural environments. (See the text of the law at https://files.eric.ed.gov/fulltext/ED433668.pdf.)

Interpretation of this law varied around the country, but essentially services moved out of the clinics and into homes, with families playing a primary role in service delivery. These changes resulted in a major shift in roles and responsibilities of practitioners. Practitioners were required to recognize family needs and desires, and to offer support to caregivers so that treatment could be integrated into the family's daily routines and activities (Campbell et al., 2009; Dunst et al., 2000; Hanft et al., 2004, 2020; McWilliam, 2010a; Sandall et al., 2005; Wilcox & Woods, 2011). This important shift acknowledged and emphasized caregivers as the experts on their children and urged practitioners to partner with families in creating intervention goals. Furthermore, the mandate recognized that learning takes place throughout the day in the context of natural relationships and that families and caregivers can be agents of change for their children.

Increased Focus on Allying With Families

Part C coincided with work and advocacy by the famous pediatrician, T. Barry Brazelton (1992), who sparked a movement among professionals to join with caregivers as allies in providing the best care for children. Brazelton urged practitioners, including his own colleagues, to move away from approaches that were "too often crisis-driven and deficit-oriented," and with caregivers' guidance, embrace children's and families' strengths (1992, p. S6).

As Part C evolved (IDEA 2004, 2011), this attitude was adopted widely. Requirements for individualized family service plans (IFSPs) shifted. The role of a service coordinator was introduced as a single point of contact for families. The service coordinator (called by many names, e.g., family resource coordinator) represented professionals from a variety of disciplines (minimally an SLP, OT, PT, and early childhood educator) and was charged with discussing recommendations made by ISFP team members with families. This single service coordinator functioned to streamline communication among the family members and other members of the family's team. The families now were seen as major partners in planning and implementing their children's therapy.

Emergence of Transdisciplinary Teams With a Primary Service Provider

Although these basic requirements for services were interpreted slightly differently by each state, one model seems to capture the current approach to service delivery for infants and toddlers: a transdisciplinary team with a PSP. The PSP, who may or may not be the service coordinator, collaborates with the family in setting IFSP goals and supporting the family in reaching these goals. This process recognizes that the parent's expertise is as important as the practitioner's. In this PSP approach, professionals from a variety of disciplines work as a team to provide coordinated services that meet the needs of children with disabilities and their families. One member of the team (the PSP) is selected to partner with the family and serve as the family's liaison to other team members (King et al., 2009; Shelden & Rush, 2013). This person represents the team's collective knowledge. This PSP transdisciplinary teaming approach utilizes "natural learning environment practices as the context for intervention and coaching as the style of interaction with the important adults in the child's life" (Shelden & Rush, 2013, p. 21).

Emphasis on Routines-Based Intervention

Service delivery in the natural environment has evolved over the years, from having families prioritize goals and other planning decisions to actual caregiver implementation of intervention. The common thread to this evolution is the routines-based approach to EI (Cripe & Venn, 1997; McWilliam, 2010a; Woods, 2005; Woods et al., 2004), whereby everyday activities in the natural environment serve as the context for working with families and children. Families become the implementers of service using whatever materials (e.g., toys, other objects) are already present in the family's home. Instruction by practitioners (i.e., the appropriate professionals) is primarily done through coaching, which refers to techniques that support others in their efforts to promote child learning and development (Rush & Shelden, 2020; Shelden & Rush, 2013). Coaching, defined in this general manner, can include other teaching strategies, and this increasingly has become the case (Brown & Woods, 2015; Salisbury et al., 2018). The PSP approach to teaming and routines-based intervention has been widely adopted, though, of course, differences in terminology, definitions, and implementation exist across programs and providers around the country. Regardless of exactly how this approach is executed, families are considered an integral part of the team and are critical for bringing about change (Bruder, 2000; Guralnick, 2001; King et al., 2009). See the following resources for more about this approach:

- See Shelden and Rush (2013) for a detailed description of the PSP approach to teaming.

- See McWilliam (2010a) and Evidence-Based International Early Intervention Office (n.d.) for a detailed description of the Routines-Based Model.

- See Woods (2005) and the Family Guided Routines Based Intervention (FGRBI) web site (http://fgrbi.com) for a detailed description of FGRBI.

TGI AND ITS RESEARCH EVOLVE TO MATCH BIRTH-TO-THREE SERVICE DELIVERY

Chapter 2 introduced TGI among other available evidence-based early interventions. This chapter continues the introduction of TGI, discussing how it complements early intervention mandates and principles. TGI was initially conceived in the 1990s by an SLP, when services were primarily provided in clinic-based settings and were tied to individual professions. This SLP, Dr. Gay Lloyd Pinder, co-author of this book, was working in a community-based center serving birth-to-three and older children at the time and became concerned about the challenges young children with moderate to severe physical disabilities (e.g., cerebral palsy) faced in engaging and communicating with their families. She purposefully designed a treatment to focus on increasing early conventional preverbal behaviors (e.g., gaze, gestures, vocalizations) that enabled children to engage and communicate with their families. This targeted treatment was delivered by the SLP during common, everyday early childhood routines such as playing with toys or eating snacks or meals, but treatment occurred primarily at the center. Due to the severity of the children's physical impairments, treatment was often delivered with a PT or OT ("co-treatment approach") (Pinder & Olswang, 1995; Pinder et al., 1993). This approach to TGI mirrored the way services for infants and toddlers were being delivered in the United States at that time, but as the field evolved, so did TGI and its research journey. Notable aspects of this evolution include the following:

- Exploring parents' role in the intervention

- Examining the breadth of TGI's application

- Investigating how TGI accommodated the general shift within birth-to-three services toward a PSP transdisciplinary teaming approach

The discussion that follows briefly describes these changes in TGI over the years. To enhance this discussion, research that was introduced in Chapter 2 is revisited, highlighting the results as they fit into the evolving birth-to-three environment.

Parents' Role in the Intervention Shifts

As TGI evolved, the role of parents shifted as they became active participants in the treatment administration. Because TGI initially had been delivered in clinic settings by an SLP, an experimental study was completed to examine the outcomes of teaching three parents to learn a treatment designed to focus on early preverbal communication behaviors (Olswang et al., 2006). Dr. Pinder taught the parents how to give their children, who exhibited moderate to severe impairments, opportunities to communicate; recognize their communicative attempts; and shape more sophisticated, conventional forms, particularly triadic gaze. Instruction occurred in the clinic setting, with suggestions on how to apply the treatment at home during play and mealtime. The study revealed that parents could successfully learn the treatment, and in turn, their children produced clearer and more recognizable preverbal communication behaviors. A side benefit of learning the TGI strategy was that the parents expressed their satisfaction and excitement in interacting with their children, particularly during toy play situations.

Breadth of TGI's Application Expands

The emerging promise of TGI to facilitate engagement and early communication increased the research teams' interest in moving it into practice. However, first research was needed to examine the training of SLPs with differences in experience and the efficacy of TGI with a larger number and greater variety of children. The training component required that the treatment protocol be tightened, thus resulting in the six-element PoWRRS-Connect protocol. This research utilized a randomized controlled study to examine preverbal communication outcomes for young children with a variety of diagnoses and an array of moderate to severe disabilities enrolled in one of two conditions: TGI condition using the PoWRRS-Connect protocol versus standard-of-care condition (Olswang et al., 2014). The PoWRRS-Connect protocol was administered by three different SLPs who had been trained to competency in delivery of the protocol in children's homes. The results demonstrated that the protocol could be successfully delivered by SLPs with different backgrounds and in natural environments. Furthermore, children enrolled in the TGI condition were more successful in becoming intentional communicators, as indicated by triadic gaze productions, than children enrolled in the standard of care condition. These promising results argued for the breadth of TGI's efficacy. This outcome, along with overall changes in service delivery for infants and toddlers, steered the research team toward their next step in evaluating and improving TGI: exploring the application of TGI in home-based service delivery settings.

TGI Accommodates the Primary Service Provider Transdisciplinary Teaming Approach

As discussed previously, birth-to-three services became more family oriented, appreciating the different types of expertise offered by caregivers versus professionals. The TGI team understood that interventions were being delivered within natural, authentic routines throughout the day by caregivers. Furthermore, the team recognized the role of transdisciplinary teams and PSPs in working with families to plan and carry out IFSPs. Investigating TGI in this context was a critical step in its evolution. The research that followed involved formalizing training via the development of a training manual for a variety of practitioners who work with infants and toddlers (i.e., SLPs, OTs, PTs). This manual included background information about emerging engagement and communication in development, the importance of focusing this aspect of development in service delivery, and a detailed explanation about the PoWRRS-Connect protocol. The emphasis of this research was on examining the practitioners' accuracy and quality of delivering the essential elements of PoWRRS-Connect, along with exploring their perceptions of the usability of TGI in their practices (Feuerstein et al., 2017, 2018). This research provided insight into the training manual, which has been incorporated into this book, and documented the success of practitioners from different backgrounds and different experiences in learning the protocol. The research also revealed the practitioners' beliefs that TGI was an important part of service delivery and that the PoWRRS-Connect protocol could be easily administered in the context of birth-to-three service delivery. Their enthusiasm for TGI in the current environment was a crucial motivation for continued analysis of the intervention and the writing of this book. Chapter 4, which will describe the application of TGI in birth-to-three services, will highlight some of the practitioners' perceptions.

The Focus of TGI Prevails

Throughout the years and the evolution of service delivery models and TGI, the focus of TGI did not change. As TGI was conceived, it is a strategy that emphasizes early engagement and children's production of early preverbal signals of communication. The evidence gathered over the years has reinforced the value of this focus while also supporting the flexibility of TGI delivery as the broader field of birth-to-three services has changed. The value of increasing children's repertoire of conventional, readable signals of communication has clearly been shown to enhance engagement with others during all types of everyday routines. What is important to understand here is that TGI emphasizes adult–child engagement and communication through a protocol designed to increase particular preverbal child behaviors, and that protocol absolutely fits into the current environment of birth-to-three services.

TGI TODAY

TGI today is an evidence-based strategy for addressing successful early engagement and communication. It adheres to the early intervention principles created by the American Speech-Language-Hearing Association (ASHA) and federal Part C requirements yet is flexible enough to be used for a variety of IFSP goals and within a variety of routines. This book addresses implementation and practical applications of TGI in service delivery for infants and toddlers, including the potential impact of the COVID-19 pandemic on implementation.

TGI, as described in this book, is implemented within the structure of ASHA's (2008a, 2008b, 2008c, 2008d) guiding principles for early intervention. These principles encompass the current Part C federal requirements and become the umbrella for TGI implementation:

- Services are family centered and culturally and linguistically responsive.

- Services are developmentally supportive and promote children's participation in their natural environments.

- Services are comprehensive, coordinated, and team based.

- Services are based on the highest quality of evidence available.

TGI is family centered, recognizing the concerns, preferences, priorities, strengths, and resources of each family and child (Paul & Roth, 2011), and embracing the families as partners in planning and delivering TGI under the guidance of the professional providing services. TGI utilizes families' knowledge and recognizes their concerns and priorities throughout service delivery. It promotes families' efforts to actively support their children's participation in daily routines and activities. TGI also appreciates that families differ, and thus the protocol can be modified to accommodate individual children's and families' styles, preferences, and cultural backgrounds (as will be explained). TGI is based on solid developmental evidence as described previously in this chapter and Chapter 2. To be specific, TGI is designed to promote children's engagement and communication with others in natural environments, and thus it is implemented in the natural environment. TGI is routines based; its PoWRRS-Connect protocol fits appropriately and naturally into everyday activities. TGI is ideally delivered as part of comprehensive, coordinated services. It can accommodate the needs of children with different types of disabilities (e.g., motor, cognitive, sensory) and degrees of severity. Furthermore, TGI and its PoWRRS-Connect protocol have been designed for transdisciplinary teams, with service providers from any of a variety of disciplines. Finally, TGI is evidence based as documented by research that occurred over nearly three decades. Table 3.1 provides a summary of principles for birth-to-three service delivery as defined by ASHA and the ways in which TGI addresses these principles.

The Part C federal regulations and ASHA principles described previously guide practitioners in service delivery. Yet, this guidance is open to different interpretations across states and agencies. Even within this diversity, TGI remains a steadfast, evidence-based strategy for addressing a fundamental need in all families: successful early engagement and communication. As will become clear in later chapters, TGI is meant to serve as a strategy for achieving a variety of IFSP goals that encompass this fundamental need. As practitioners support and coach families during daily routines, they must have in their toolbox a variety of strategies for assisting families in building their capacity to help their children successfully participate in everyday activities. TGI can be one of those strategies. Practitioners should consider TGI as an evidence-based strategy that serves to enhance caregivers' skills and abilities for building their children's intentional communication signals, which in turn will result in increased and satisfying interactions. TGI and its PoWRRS-Connect protocol

Table 3.1. Summary of principles for birth-to-three service delivery and how Triadic Gaze Intervention (TGI) addresses them

The match between birth-to-three service delivery principles and TGI	
Guiding principles for birth-to-three service delivery*	TGI application
Family-centered services are culturally and linguistically responsive.	TGI embraces families as partners. It values families' knowledge. It recognizes families' concerns and priorities. It recognizes differences in beliefs, practices, and priorities across families.
Services are developmentally supportive and promote children's participation in their natural environments.	TGI promotes early preverbal communication behaviors (i.e., gaze, gestures, vocalizations) that have been well documented in research. It promotes children's engagement and communication in the natural environment. It fits into families' everyday routines.
Services are comprehensive, coordinated, and team based.	TGI accommodates children with a variety of disabilities and characteristics that are best served by a transdisciplinary team.
Services are based on the highest quality of evidence available.	TGI is evidence based, resulting from research across three decades, including feasibility, randomized controlled, and implementation studies.

*Based on guidelines from the American Speech-Language-Hearing Association (ASHA, 2008a, 2008b, 2008c, 2008d).

have flexible application to meet the individual needs of children and their families, and for seamless use across a variety of daily routines. As the PoWRRS-Connect protocol is described in detail in Chapters 5, 6, and 7, practitioners will be urged to consider its extensive and practical application across IFSP goals and families' varied activities.

CONCLUSION

Birth-to-three services and TGI have evolved to accommodate fundamental ideas and wisdom about the content and form of service delivery for very young children with moderate to severe disabilities and their families. Valuing and utilizing parent expertise, appreciating the importance of transdisciplinary teams, and understanding that maximum learning occurs in natural environments in the context of authentic routines have all been incorporated into services for infants and toddlers. This chapter has explored this evolution and discussed its impact on TGI, including how the research evidence followed and addressed the various changes. TGI as it is described in this book matches the current principles and guidelines for birth-to-three services. No doubt delivery of these services will continue to evolve as times change and knowledge expands. TGI's adaptability should make it a resilient strategy for building the all-important development of engagement and communication. Chapter 4 will provide an overview of TGI, delineating the essential elements of its PoWRRS-Connect protocol, and will further explain its value to practitioners and families of children with moderate to severe disabilities.

Implementing Triadic Gaze Intervention

CHAPTER **4**

Introduction to the Triadic Gaze Intervention

What, Who, Where, When, and Why

This chapter introduces the reader to the core features of TGI. It serves as an overview to describe the purpose of TGI, the essential elements composing the treatment protocol (PoWRRS-Connect), and the delivery of the protocol (who, where, and when). This overview chapter is meant to introduce—not teach—the essential elements of PoWRRS-Connect and, as such, provide the reader with a broad sense of the protocol and how it is meant to be implemented throughout the day during naturally occurring activities and **authentic routines**. To illustrate how practitioners feel about the implementation of TGI, quotations capturing their perceptions of the protocol are scattered throughout the chapter (from Feuerstein et al., 2018). The chapter ends with a summary that highlights the value of TGI and provides a case for its use. Subsequent chapters will go into detail about the protocol itself and how it is used in practice.

WHAT IS THE PURPOSE OF TGI?

TGI is a strategy practitioners can employ to help families engage and communicate with their young children with disabilities. All parents want their children to talk; yet, so much happens before talking. Development of language in any form (spoken words, signs, or augmentative and alternative communication) relies on a foundation of skills that allows for positive interactions with others. For children with disabilities, these foundational skills are often limited. Families might say they have trouble understanding what their children want or need, or they might say it is hard to interact or play with their children. The overall goal of TGI is to increase the ease with which families interact with their children by helping them recognize their children's communication attempts and increase their children's repertoire of conventional communication signals. The PoWRRS-Connect protocol is the implementation arm of TGI; it is designed to facilitate the production of gaze, gestures, and vocalizations that lead to triadic gaze as a readable signal of intentional communication. However, do not assume TGI is just about skill development; it is not. TGI is a strategy practitioners can introduce to families for emphasizing and encouraging preverbal connections. It is a strategy that builds children's readable signals within the context of the families' guidance. Moreover, TGI is a strategy that emphasizes interactions throughout the day, and as a result, can become a part of families' typical, authentic routines. The implementation of TGI through PoWRRS-Connect will fit into a variety of activities and experiences, including pure social engagement, play with toys, and functional routines (e.g., mealtime, bath time). Simply put, TGI highlights the importance of engagement and communication and becomes a strategy for enabling families to encourage their children with disabilities to become active participants in their world.

WHAT IS THE TGI STRATEGY?

TGI is a strategy that recognizes the importance of engagement and communication as part of birth-to-three services for children with disabilities and complex communication needs (CCNs). TGI emphasizes connections between children and others and prioritizes the facilitation of intentional communication via preverbal behaviors of gaze, gestures, and vocalizations. TGI acknowledges that a lot of communication happens prior to children's producing first words. TGI is realized through the implementation of a six-element protocol (acronym **PoWRRS-Connect**) designed to facilitate the production of early communication behaviors. The six essential elements will feel familiar, as they correspond to the components of a typical adult–child turn-taking interaction. We hope the acronym will assist practitioners and caregivers in remembering the six elements:

> Practitioners have noted that TGI increased their awareness of early preverbal communication in delivering early supports: "I feel like it's already changed the way that we're doing treatment. It's already helped give me more of a focus."
>
> On the importance of gaze, a practitioner noted: ". . . [the child] has to connect to communicate with you. He has to look at you" and ". . . while the aim was to work on his eye gaze and communication, we've seen a big improvement in how he's been able to play and interact and be involved more."
>
> (Feuerstein et al., 2018)

1. Structure the environment to **provide an opportunity (Po)** for engagement and communication.

2. **Wait (PoW)** for a child to produce a potentially communicative behavior.

3. **Recognize (PoWR)** and

4. **Respond (PoWRR)** to the child's behavior.

5. **Shape (PoWRRS)** that behavior to a more readable, conventional signal (ultimately, triadic gaze).

6. **Connect (PoWRRS-Connect)** with the child in an appropriate manner, to reinforce the child's efforts.

The six elements are administered in a semi-structured manner, typically involving the adult, child, and an object, and are best conceived as a cyclical flow starting with a natural connection and ending with that natural connection resuming. Figure 4.1 illustrates

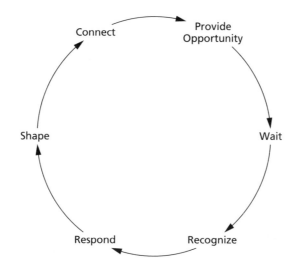

Figure 4.1.   PoWRRS-Connect six-element protocol envisioned as a cycle.

the cycle in which the six essential elements of PoWRRS-Connect protocol should be delivered. The cycle can be implemented multiple times a day across a variety of settings and situations.

Before breaking down each of the elements, consider this typical scenario: Mother and child are playing with bubbles. The mother blows the bubbles and the child watches them, giggling and making sounds of delight. The mother repeats blowing the bubbles and eventually starts popping them, one at a time. The child laughs and tries to reach up toward the bubbles. The mother continues the game. In TGI, this reflects the *connection* that is occurring between the adult and child. In our scenario, the mother then pauses blowing the bubbles and says to the child, "Do you want more?" She is *providing an opportunity in the form of a request*. The mother then *waits and watches* the child for a signal that the child wants more or is done with the game. The child starts to laugh, puckers the lips (perhaps as if blowing), and squeals as they are looking at their mother. The mother *recognizes* these behaviors and *responds* to them by saying to the child, "You want more bubbles, don't you." She then shakes the bubble jar, saying, "More bubbles," which gets her child to look at the jar, thus shaping a new behavior of looking at adult and object. The mother smiles and says, "Wow, you're looking at the bubbles; you must want more of those bubbles" and proceeds to blow the bubbles again, resuming the game. This whole activity will no doubt occur again and again—until the mother or the child gets tired of it and they are ready to move on to the next activity. In this one activity, the bubble game, the PoWRRS-Connect protocol can be implemented many times, thus providing many occasions for engaging and communicating, reinforcing, and teaching signals of communication. We turn now to defining each element in the PoWRRS-Connect TGI protocol.

WHAT ELEMENTS MAKE UP THE PoWRRS-CONNECT PROTOCOL?

The six essential elements of the PoWRRS-Connect protocol are highlighted in Table 4.1 and introduced in the sections that follow.

Table 4.1. Six essential elements of PoWRRS-Connect

1. Provide opportunity (Po)	Structure the environment to engage the child and give them a chance to communicate.
2. Wait (W)	Give the child time to produce a communicative behavior.
3. Recognize (R)	Acknowledge the child's attempt to communicate, whatever the form.
4. Respond (R)	Interpret the child's behavior.
5. Shape (S)	When appropriate, help the child perform a communicative behavior that is just beyond their capacity by using a variety of prompts.
6. Connect (C)	Interact with the child to reinforce the child's participation.

Provide Opportunity

Providing an opportunity occurs during an ongoing interaction and refers to setting up a clear occasion for engaging and communicating with the child. Clear occasion defines the Provide opportunity (Po). TGI encourages request and choice opportunities during social or functional interactions as they provide clear, almost obligatory opportunities for a child to communicate and exert control over their world. **Request opportunities** can include requesting an object out of reach or requesting more of an action that was paused (e.g., requesting more bubble blowing, "Do you want more bubbles?"). **Choice opportunities** include offering the child a choice between two toys held before them (e.g., "Do you want the ball or the bubbles?"). The essence of this element is that it breaks up the flow of an ongoing interaction and provides an obvious chance for the child to communicate. **Commenting opportunities** are also useful but not obligatory for the child to participate. For example, the adult might make an animated comment (e.g., "Oh look! Wow! That's a big dog"), then look with anticipation at the child. The purpose of the Po element is to encourage a child's involvement during an interaction and provide a clear occasion for them to communicate; it passes the turn to the child.

Wait (PoW)

Waiting refers to giving the child time to produce some engaged and communicative behavior following the presentation of an opportunity (request, choice, or comment). Waiting is essential to give the child time to show their best effort. For children with disabilities, this is particularly important.

Recognize (PoWR)

Following the presentation of the communication opportunity and waiting, the child will do something that the adult needs to recognize. The child can show a variety of behaviors, clear or subtle, requiring the adult to be sensitive to what the child is bringing to the interaction as well as their intent. These behaviors might communicate "more" or a choice, a comment, or even possibly a protest. A child might produce one or more of the behaviors along the communication behavioral continuum: single focus, dual focus, and/or triadic gaze with or without gestures and vocalizations (e.g., looking at the ball or the bubbles). As an alternative, the child might produce idiosyncratic behaviors (e.g., lifting a finger to comment, extending their body to request, squirming away and fussing as a protest). The focus is on recognizing whatever behavior the child is producing or trying to produce. Practitioners and caregivers will need to work together to identify unconventional behaviors that have the potential to be communicative.

Respond (PoWRR)

Once the adult has recognized the child's attempt to communicate and interpreted its meaning, the adult needs to respond to this effort. This means acknowledging the behavior by naming it (e.g., "Oh, you looked at the ball") and then appropriately responding to the child's intention (e.g., "Okay, here's the ball," giving it to the child).

Shape (PoWRRS)

Because TGI is designed to facilitate the child's production of new, more readable communicative behaviors, the shaping element is particularly important. Shaping means helping the child successfully perform a behavior or task that is just beyond their capacity but is developmentally appropriate. Another term for shaping that is used professionally is scaffolding. This is accomplished by structuring the context so that the child can gradually move from performing where they are comfortable to successfully performing a new, challenging behavior or task within reach. Shaping involves providing verbal, visual, auditory, and/or tactile **prompts** to support a child's performance of a more sophisticated, conventional communicative behavior. In TGI, the triadic gaze behavior with or without gestures and vocalizations is the ultimate goal as a signal of intentional communication. The prompts to shape are selected to match individual children's preferences for teaching. Shaping is an exciting part of the protocol but is often viewed as the most difficult to implement. Once the child tries to produce the new behavior, the adult will reinforce the child's attempt, regardless of whether it is successful. This will include describing the child's attempt (e.g., "Oh, you tried to look at me and the ball") and, of course, fulfilling the communicative attempt (e.g., giving the child the ball). Again, practitioners will need to work closely with families to determine when it is appropriate to shape, what behaviors are most suitable to attempt, and the types of prompts that seem most useful.

Connect (PoWRRS-Connect)

Every communication opportunity ends by supporting the child's connection with the adult, and when an object or toy is involved, exploring and manipulating the toy the child has requested, chosen, or commented on. Thus, connect at the end of the cycle serves three main goals: 1) to reinforce the child's communication attempt, 2) to demonstrate the power of communication, and 3) when involving a toy or object, to expose the child to various ways to explore and manipulate toys. The type of connection that follows each opportunity also provides the context for setting up the next opportunity to engage and communicate. This cycle can continue over and over throughout an activity. When playing with toys, different toys can be introduced in a series of choice and request opportunities. Object play situations are encouraged because they are ideal for demonstrating to the child how the adult can serve as a means to an end and for reinforcing a child's sense of agency (i.e., directing others' actions).

WHO DELIVERS THE PoWRRS-CONNECT PROTOCOL?

TGI is a strategy for use in the natural environment and, as such, is compatible with the transdisciplinary, PSP, and routines-based models and other similar approaches to birth-to-three support services. Implementation of TGI relies on the partnership between practitioners and families. This partnership is crucial to the success of TGI as an early support strategy. The practitioner serves as the coach to the families, bringing their expertise in child development and disabilities to the partnership. TGI offers guidance to the practitioner about the specific skills and knowledge that are necessary for children and their families as they build successful and enjoyable social interactions. The families bring expertise about their children and home environment to the partnership. The families are essential for planning how to best use the TGI strategy, and specifically the PoWRRS-Connect protocol, during daily routines (e.g., identifying child preferences for materials and family activities). As such, TGI offers a guide for practitioners in coaching parents to help their children produce readable behaviors of communication (gaze, gestures, and vocalizations) during interactions throughout the day.

Early support services often use the PSP model, which requires that the team choose one member to work with the family while getting input from the other team members. That member typically is chosen based on the family's area of primary concern and the focus of referral. This focus may be motor development, early feeding issues, cognition, or another area of concern. When the child is an infant or toddler (6–18 months) who has more severe disabilities and is seeking early support services, the referrals are often based on early motor or feeding concerns but rarely based on concerns in the area of early communication. This is most likely because both pediatricians and families are primarily focused on addressing motor and feeding worries; communication often is not even under consideration because children do not typically talk or produce first words until approximately 12–15 months. Thus, the initial PSP is most likely to be the PT or OT, unless the SLP has skills in addressing early feeding issues. This is unfortunate as a tremendous amount of communication occurs prior to first words. The gift of the SLP is that they can bring to early support services an extensive knowledge of early preverbal communication development, from preintentional to intentional gaze, gestures, and vocalizations. The SLP is trained to set up communication opportunities and to facilitate and recognize a child's communicative behaviors, including subtle ones. The SLP's perspective dovetails perfectly with the PT's or OT's knowledge of motor and sensory development; together, they offer a family a holistic picture of the child. Working with the PT or OT, the SLP can help the family recognize the child's communication attempts and then, through the family routines, such as play, snack time, bath, and bedtime, expand and enrich the effectiveness and depth of the communication.

Because of TGI's focus, support teams are urged to include an SLP to provide insights about early preverbal development of communication. Although SLPs will be valuable for tailoring TGI and the PoWRRS-Connect protocol to individual families, as noted previously, the strategy was designed for use by practitioners from any discipline

> One practitioner noted: "We come, and we provide support; the parent is the expert on the child."
>
> Practitioners see themselves as respectfully guiding parents: "You have to consider both the child's needs and what the parents are capable of, or what they want for their child . . . and kind of follow their lead, but also educate them on what the possibilities are for their child, and how their child can get there. And then let them decide."
>
> (Feuerstein et al., 2018)

that supports infants and toddlers. Appropriateness of TGI for a child and their family will be determined through conventional evaluation and assessment procedures that qualify a child for services and determine child and family needs and priorities. Success of the TGI strategy will rely on the strength of the practitioner–family partnership: practitioner as coach and family as implementer.

One final thought about who delivers TGI: The importance of the caregiver–practitioner partnership cannot be overstated. The practitioner is the guide and the caregiver the implementer. Is it possible to deliver TGI via telehealth service delivery? Yes. As the year 2020 demonstrated, birth-to-three service delivery may need to be packaged in different forms, including via online platforms. Practitioners have gained tremendous skills in accommodating to this reality. Although TGI was developed for in-person delivery, it can be adapted for a variety of telehealth models. The success will depend on the practitioner and caregiver working together as they would in implementing any intervention.

WHERE AND WHEN IS PoWRRS-CONNECT DELIVERED?

PoWRRS-Connect ideally is delivered in the home, during routine activities, by the family. Interactions between families and children occur all day long. Some interactions are more social, involving the adult and child being together for moments of comfort or play, such as playing Peekaboo. Other interactions are more functional, such as those that take place during mealtime, bath time, or toy or object play. Either kind of interaction can involve a variety of nonverbal communicative intentions on the part of the adult and child (i.e., either adult or child initiated): most commonly, protesting, requesting (actions, objects, and information), commenting (on actions and objects), and answering.

Requesting and choosing are particularly valuable for eliciting and observing children's communicative attempts, and for demonstrating the power of their behaviors. During these interactions, children are engaging with the adult to get help or assistance; as such, the situations typically involve the triad of adult, child, and object. Consider, for example, the saliency of the following communicative interactions that take place during mealtime: The child indicates they want more juice or is asked to choose between a cracker and banana. Or consider social play between a child and favorite person, where the adult is making funny noises to entertain the child, stopping every few seconds to see if the child wants more (i.e., a request). These contexts lend themselves to setting up clear opportunities for engaging and communicating, observing child communicative attempts, acknowledging the child's participation, and introducing new behaviors to the child, as occurs in PoWRRS-Connect. Request and choice are salient social and functional interactions that adults can construct to increase the likelihood of a child's participation and engagement. They tend to be dominant during everyday activities. Note particularly that requesting and choosing typically involve objects, and recall that children with disabilities are often limited in exposure to objects or toys. Thus, these contexts become valuable for observing, eliciting, and teaching communication skills and for facilitating knowledge of objects and object relations, through encouraging attainment and manipulation of toys.

As children learn that they can effectively express their wants and needs, they begin to understand that they have agency and can direct the actions of others. This is critical for all children, but imagine how important this understanding is for children with disabilities who are challenged in physically acting on their world. How magnificent for these children to learn that they have some control over their environment! The PoWRRS-Connect protocol utilizes requesting and choosing during social and functional interactions to a great extent because of these qualities. This is not to say that other communicative intentions (e.g., commenting on actions or objects, answering, protesting) do not provide opportunities for engaging and communicating; they certainly do. Adults should always be on the lookout for any moment where a child is trying to engage and share. Because details about PoWRRS-Connect are further explained in subsequent chapters, they will address these other types of opportunities.

> Practitioners noted:
> "It fits in every way. It's easy to teach parents. It's empowering for parents. It can happen in a natural environment. It can be taught. It can be coached. It can be modeled."
> "I've been surprised at how easy it is to teach this to parents and to have them embed it. They don't have to buy anything. It makes sense to them."
> "Caregivers ran with it—whatever part that resonated with them."
> (Feuerstein et al., 2018)

WHY USE TRIADIC GAZE INTERVENTION?

The clear value of TGI lies in its purpose and its practical application. The following points highlight the unique and appealing features of the TGI strategy:

- Emphasizes engagement and communication in birth-to-three services.

- Establishes early preverbal behaviors that are foundational to language of any form (spoken words, signs, or augmentative and alternative communication symbols).

- Emphasizes intentional communication through triadic gaze as a building block for future cognitive, social, and language development.

- Builds successful engagement and communication between families and their children with disabilities.

- Encourages positive social interactions and exposure to a variety of play activities.

- Provides a straightforward structure for application in the context of everyday, authentic routines and activities.

- Consists of a six-element PoWRRS-Connect protocol that mirrors the logical and familiar components of any turn-taking interaction.

- Breaks down the task of communicating into smaller, more manageable parts, which provides an ideal context for learning but does not interfere with how interactions occur typically.

- Makes something easier that might otherwise be difficult for some children with disabilities and their families.

- Can be employed in a variety of IFSP goals.

TGI is a strategy that emphasizes encouraging engagement and communication between children with disabilities and their families. It helps build successful social relationships and boosts independence for children who exhibit challenges across developmental domains. TGI provides a strategy particularly suited for addressing and overcoming these challenges by facilitating children's production of more conventional and readable preverbal communication behaviors. For children who have difficulty expressing their wants and needs, TGI may be an appropriate strategy to offer families.

CONCLUSION

This chapter has emphasized the value of TGI for children with CCN and their families. It is viewed as a strategy that practitioners can employ as they coach families during activities designed to address IFSP goals. TGI is implemented through six essential elements abbreviated as PoWRRS-Connect; this protocol is straightforward in breaking down an interaction between an adult and a child. It emphasizes the individual elements of turn taking, which ensures engagement and offers an ideal context for learning how to communicate. It is meant to encourage the production of conventional preverbal communication behaviors (ultimately, triadic gaze) that will be recognized and reinforced by others. Through the application of PoWRRS-Connect throughout the day, during a variety of routine activities, TGI can build connections between children and others. It ultimately allows for exchanges that can provide a foundation for all kinds of learning. Some children and families certainly will seem suited for TGI, and others will not. The next chapter explores the process of considering whether TGI is appropriate for a child and their family, and how TGI will fit into IFSP planning.

CHAPTER 5

Integrating Triadic Gaze Intervention Into Practice

Determining the Appropriateness of TGI for Children and Families

TGI is one strategy that can be used to support children's early communication skills and engagement with others and their world. But how do you know which children and families may benefit from TGI? This chapter is designed to help practitioners determine if TGI is a good fit to support a family in achieving their goals and objectives for their child.

The chapter is organized around the standard process used throughout the country for qualifying and enrolling children and families in Part C services. This process, depicted in Figure 5.1, includes the initial referral, intake, evaluation and assessment, and IFSP development, which then leads to service delivery. The Early Childhood Technical Assistance Center (ECTA, 2014) has created a document providing a detailed overview of this process, currently available at the ECTA web site at https://ectacenter.org/eco/assets/pdfs/IFSP-OutcomesFlowChart.pdf. This chapter describes how birth-to-three teams can gather information during each step in this process to determine if TGI might be useful as part of services for particular children and families.

IS TGI A GOOD FIT FOR CHILDREN AND FAMILIES?

The process of determining if TGI is a good fit for a child and family should complement the processes and procedures already used by agencies around the country for determining services for infants and toddlers. Consideration of the appropriateness of TGI for a child and family will start at the beginning of the process: the initial referral.

INITIAL REFERRAL

Certain child characteristics noted at the time of referral may suggest to the team members that they should be considering TGI. These characteristics include the child being between 10 and 36 months old and exhibiting moderate to severe disabilities that affect sensory, motor, cognitive, and/or social-emotional development. As a result of these

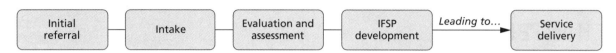

Figure 5.1. The early intervention process, from referral to service delivery. (*Key:* IFSP, individualized family service plan.)

developmental disabilities, children's communication skills will be limited, which will be indicated by the absence of identifiable words, word approximations, or signs. Children will be described by families as having difficulty engaging with others and making their wants and needs clearly known. These child characteristics are listed in Table 5.1 and are based on criteria used in past TGI research protocols. (See Appendix A for a summary of this research program.)

When a child presents with these characteristics, TGI may be an appropriate strategy for building early communication competence and engaged interactions with caregivers. The next steps in the process serve to further clarify the child's strengths and areas of need as well as the family's priorities. These steps will give additional information that helps the team determine the appropriateness of TGI.

INTAKE

Following referral, an intake is scheduled, by phone or in person. Intake typically will be conducted by a service coordinator, who provides the family with information about early intervention services in their area. That service coordinator may also perform a developmental screening, depending on the guidelines of that area. If the family consents to an evaluation and assessment, the service coordinator then gathers important demographic information, obtains relevant medical records or other reports, and learns about the family's general concerns and priorities. This intake material, which is shared with the team for assessment planning, should trigger thinking about whether TGI may be appropriate. Some specific questions that may be asked during intake include:

- Does your child have an established medical condition that results in disabilities affecting sensory, motor, cognitive, and/or social-emotional development?

- Does your child have difficulty engaging during games such as Peekaboo, singing songs, or other social interactions?

Table 5.1. Child characteristics that suggest Triadic Gaze Intervention may be a good fit

Age	Overall development	Communication skills
10–36 months	Moderate to severe disabilities affecting • Sensory development • Motor development • Cognitive development • Social-emotional development	• Not yet producing any identifiable words, word approximations, or signs • Experiencing challenges in making wants and needs known • Having difficulty engaging with caregivers in social interactions

- Does your child have difficulty communicating their wants and needs using facial expressions, gestures, or sounds/word approximations?

- Does your child have difficulty playing with toys on their own?

If a family answers yes to any of these questions, the service coordinator may alert the team that TGI might be appropriate. Consider the following vignette.

Intake: Matthew, Age 18 Months

The service coordinator receives a referral for Matthew, an 18-month-old boy with Down syndrome. The referral, faxed from the family's pediatrician, requests an evaluation for physical therapy services, highlighting hypotonia and the potential need for adaptive seating equipment. The service coordinator notes that the pediatrician's primary concern is about Matthew's motor skills, but during the intake phone call with the family, she asks, "Does Matthew have any difficulty communicating what he wants or needs?" She quickly learns that the family has concerns about Matthew's ability to communicate. The family reports that they have trouble determining what he wants, and they do a lot of guessing. Matthew doesn't make eye contact and becomes frustrated when they do not understand him. The family reports that Matthew will throw toys or bat them away and even bite and scratch when his siblings do not understand him. Although the pediatrician has picked up on the motor delay, the family is also concerned about the possibility of a delay in Matthew's communication skills. Given this child's profile and the family concerns, the service coordinator flags the file as a potential fit for TGI, which may help give Matthew a way to successfully communicate with family members and reduce the frustration Matthew is feeling.

EVALUATION AND ASSESSMENT

Following intake, family consent is obtained for the child evaluation and assessment. At this visit, the team 1) evaluates the child's skills and abilities to determine eligibility for Part C services and 2) assesses and documents the child's developing strengths and challenges, as well as family strengths and challenges during daily routines (Individuals with Disabilities Education Act [IDEA] of 2004, PL 108-446). Each of these steps provides an opportunity to engage with families in conversation about the purpose and appropriateness of TGI.

Evaluation

A multidisciplinary evaluation typically will be conducted to determine if a child qualifies for Part C services in their state. Children qualify for these services by either 1) having an established medical condition or 2) meeting a predetermined criterion for having developmental delay, which varies state by state. The Early Childhood Technical Assistance Center has published a document that outlines eligibility criteria for Part C services across the United States, currently available at the ECTA (2015) web site.

The initial evaluation to determine a child's eligibility for Part C services typically utilizes standardized tests to address five developmental domains: cognitive, physical (fine and gross motor), communication, self-help/adaptive behavior, and social-emotional skills. Although specific evaluation tools used by agencies or providers will vary within and across states, the information obtained from the initial child evaluation will help identify the child's developmental strengths and challenges and will assist the team and the family to begin thinking about which early intervention services will be appropriate to meet child and family needs. A thorough developmental evaluation will include details about a child's engagement and early communication skills, regardless of the tests or tools used to conduct the evaluation.

The team is encouraged to consider the child's performance on the evaluation when thinking about the appropriateness of TGI for a child and family. Much information about a child's communication and engagement skills can be gained from the test and tools that are already used as part of the evaluation process. For example, if parent report tools are used, such as The Rossetti Infant-Toddler Language Scale (Rossetti, 2006), the team can note how parents respond to specific items that target early communication or engagement. Likewise, if direct evaluation of a child's skills is used, such as the Bayley Scales of Infant and Toddler Development (Bayley, 2009), the team can elicit and document how a child performs on specific test items that target early communication or social engagement behaviors.

Table 5.2 presents a list of communication and engagement behaviors that are foundational for triadic gaze production and offers examples of items from two commonly used tests, The Rossetti Infant-Toddler Language Scale (Rossetti, 2006) and DAYC-2, Developmental Assessment of Young Children – Second Edition (Voress et al., 2012), that help determine which foundational behaviors the child already has in their repertoire. Note that the list of examples is not exhaustive but is provided to give assessment teams a point from which to start understanding the rich information that they are gathering during the evaluation, which might be informative when considering the application of TGI. Other commonly used assessments, such as the Preschool Language Scales 5th Edition (Zimmerman, Steiner, & Pond, 2011) and Bayley Scales of Infant and Toddler Development

Table 5.2.   Communication and engagement behaviors foundational for triadic gaze production: Examples of items from commonly used tests and tools

Communication and engagement behaviors foundational for triadic gaze	Example items (test/tool name)
Looks at or shows interest in people	• Cries to get attention (Rosetti) • Waves hi and bye (Rosetti) • Smiles at person who is talking or gesturing (DAYC-2) • Imitates familiar action after observing caregiver doing (e.g., claps hands) (DAYC-2)
Looks at or shows interest in objects	• Reaches for objects (Rosetti) • Eyes follow ball rolling (Bayley) • Looks back and forth between two objects (DAYC-2) • Explores objects in a variety of ways (DAYC-2)
Shifts gaze from object to person or person to object	• Hands object to adult to have them repeat or start a desired action (DAYC-2)
Looks back and forth between object and person	(No items found on tests or tools examined.)

Key: Rosetti, The Rossetti Infant-Toddler Language Scale (Rossetti, 2006); DAYC-2, Developmental Assessment of Young Children–Second Edition (Voress et al., 2012).

(From Rossetti, L. M. [2006]. The Rossetti Infant-Toddler Language Scale. Austin: PRO-ED. Reprinted by permission; from Voress, J., Maddox, T., & Hammill, D. [2012]. Developmental Assessment of Young Children - Second Edition [DAYC-2]. Austin: PRO-ED. Reprinted by permission.)

(Bayley, 2009), also include items addressing behaviors such as looking briefly at or vocalizing at someone who is speaking, reaching for objects or following moving objects with one's eyes, and otherwise showing interest in people or objects.

If the evaluation suggests that the child is demonstrating some of these foundational skills but is not yet using triadic gaze (looking back and forth between objects/events and people, as described in Chapter 1), then TGI may be an important strategy to build communication and engagement, as part of the child's support services. *Remember*: TGI is employed to help move children toward conventional signals of intentional communication, specifically production of triadic gaze. TGI is designed to help children produce behaviors along the communication continuum at their own pace, appreciating that they will vary in their capacity to reach triadic gaze. TGI is a strategy that presumes potential for engaging and communicating with a variety of signals. However, children who are not demonstrating any of the foundational skills noted in Table 5.2 will likely not be ready for TGI. Rather, they will need support for attaining earlier developing behaviors, for example, alerting and attending to stimuli in the environment. Such behaviors would be seen as foundational achievements for considering TGI as a strategy to employ. The next section discusses how practitioners may begin a conversation about TGI with family members and discuss its appropriateness for supporting their child's early communication development.

Assessment

Assessment is an ongoing process that occurs throughout a family's time in early intervention. Both the child and the family are the focus of assessment. Assessment typically is accomplished through detailed, ongoing conversations with the family as well as observation of the child's skills within everyday routines and activities. Assessment therefore can provide the team with additional, potentially more in-depth, information than acquired through evaluation alone. This rich information will help the team decide if TGI may be an appropriate strategy to support families in accomplishing the goals they articulate for their children. The sections that follow first discuss how the practitioner might learn more about the family's daily routines, which serve as the context for intervention, and then, more specifically, learn about the child's communication behaviors within those routines.

Family Routines as the Context for Communication and Social Engagement During the assessment process, the birth-to-three team learns about what is working well for the family (i.e., identifying the child's and family's resources, strengths, and interests) and what is challenging (i.e., identifying the family's concerns). Learning about the family's routines provides the context for understanding the child's communication and social engagement skills. This information will provide additional clues for considering the value of TGI. Some practitioners will engage the family in a formal interview; others will be less structured. Some teams may ask directly about the child's level of social interaction, engagement, and independence, using questions such as the following:

- How does the child let you know they want something?

- When you are feeding the child, how do they let you know they want more?

- How does the child say "no"?

- Do you offer the child choices? How does the child tell you which is their choice?

- How does the child protest? Does the child look at you when they are crying?

A family's answers to questions like these will shed light on whether engagement and/or communication are areas of concern.

Teams often will ask open-ended questions about the family's day-to-day life, including questions that explore the child's role in the family's everyday routines and activities (see McWilliam, 2010b, for a guide for how to conduct a routines-based interview). These types of questions might look like the following:

- Which parts of your day are going well? Which parts are difficult?

- Which routines are going well? Why?

- Which routines are challenging? Why?

- What would make these routines go more easily?

- What are the things your child enjoys the most (including toys, people, activities)?

- What do you enjoy doing with your child?

- How do you play with your child?

- What games are fun for you both?

Although family members may not state directly that they are worried about their young child's communication skills or ability to engage, the answers to these questions help describe the role communication and engagement play in their daily routines and activities. The family members' responses to these kinds of questions should get the team thinking about whether TGI could be useful. Consider the following vignettes.

Evaluation and Assessment: David, Age 16 Months

David is 16 months old and recently started to sit independently. His family was referred to their local EI agency for a developmental evaluation and assessment. The evaluation, completed by an SLP and OT, documented that David presents with delays in fine and gross motor skills, as well as in communication skills, sufficient to qualify for EI services in his area. To complete the assessment, a service coordinator visits David and his family at home. She observes David interacting with his mom and asks questions about the family's routines and David's communication skills. David is sitting near his mother. He is holding a toy but is not able to easily manipulate the toy, in part because of his precarious sitting balance but also because David's fine motor challenges make playing with the toy difficult. His frustration is clear. His mother tries to assist him while she is talking with the service coordinator. "This is when we can have trouble," she states. "He wants to play, but he wants to do it himself, and he gets frustrated when we try to help." The service coordinator asks, "When you are playing together, how does he ask for help?" His mother replies, "He doesn't. He just keeps trying to play with the toy but gets more and more frustrated. He won't even look at us! If he just weren't so stubborn . . . or if he could just talk, things would be so much easier. Even just yes and no would help!"

Evaluation and Assessment: Maya, Age 24 Months

Maya is 24 months old and has an undiagnosed syndrome with clear developmental delays in both motor skills and cognitive/play skills. A service coordinator and SLP visit Maya and her mother at home to complete an assessment before writing IFSP goals with the family. During the visit, Maya is sitting on her mom's lap playing with her hands. The service coordinator asks questions while the SLP works to engage Maya. The SLP holds several toys side by side to see if Maya will look at the toys or even reach for one. The service coordinator asks Mom, "Do you offer her choices? How does she tell you which toy she wants?" Maya's Mom replies, "Oh, I have never given her a choice. I always just hand her a toy or put it on the high-chair tray in front of her. She can't talk, so how can she tell me?"

These vignettes highlight how information gained from a conversation with a family supplements what is gathered during the more formal child evaluation that is used to qualify a child for Part C services. By asking a few simple questions, the team can learn a lot about what a family is thinking and feeling about their child's strengths and challenges. In the two vignettes, information begins to emerge that suggests engagement and communication may be a problem for the children and their families. David may be lacking early communication behaviors, specifically gaze. Maya may be experiencing limited opportunities to demonstrate her communication skills. In both cases, the team would become alerted to look further at engagement and early communication and consider TGI as part of the service plan.

The Child's Communication Behaviors   During these conversations, the team begins to learn about the quality of the social interactions between the family and the child during their everyday routines and activities. These discussions can reveal which communicative behaviors the child is producing and how easy (or not) it is for families to recognize these behaviors. Parents and caregivers are the experts on their children, but labeling the specific early communication behaviors that their child can produce (gaze, gestures, vocalizations) can be challenging. Sometimes, information about specific behaviors can come from conversations with caregivers. Other times, observing children interact with their caregivers will reveal this information. In either case, to help practitioners gather this preliminary information, a Checklist of Early Communication Behaviors is provided in Figure 5.2 and Appendix B. A downloadable, printable checklist is also available at the Brookes Download Hub with the other online resources for this book.

The Checklist of Early Communication Behaviors can be completed during assessment but also at any time prior to beginning treatment and, as will be discussed in Chapter 9, during and after treatment to measure progress. This checklist displays conventional early communication behaviors in three categories: gaze, vocalizations, and gestures. Within each category, behaviors are listed along a continuum from simple to more complex. The columns in the middle of the checklist with the header "Source of Information" provide space for practitioners to make a note of the gaze, gesture, and vocal behaviors that the child produces, including those reported by caregivers and/or

Checklist of Early Communication Behaviors

Name:

Foundational Behaviors for Triadic Gaze			Source of Information		Notes
			Caregiver Reported	Practitioner Observed	Activity or Routine, Toys or Objects, People Present, Prompts Used
Gaze	Single Focus	Looks and sustains gaze to a **person***			
		Looks and sustains gaze to an **object***			
		Follows a moving **object***			
	Dual Focus	Looks back and forth between **two objects***			
		Looks from **object to person OR person to object***			
	Triadic Focus	Looks **back and forth** between object **AND** person*			
Vocalizations		Produces **early sounds** (fusses, squeals)			
		Produces **consonants, vowels,** and **consonant–vowel combinations**			
		Produces **word approximations**			
Gestures		**Leans/reaches** for object **OR** person*			
		Shows, points, gives			
		Uses **gestures** meaningfully (waves hi/bye, covers eyes for Peekaboo)			

*NOTE: Be sure to note if the child also uses vocalizations and/or gestures when looking.

Figure 5.2. Checklist of Early Communication Behaviors.

those behaviors directly observed during the assessment. The practitioner may simply put a checkmark in the box next to the behavior that the child produces. Finally, on the far right of the checklist, there is space for the practitioner to jot down notes about observations made during the visit with the family, including information about the activity or routine observed, the child's communication partner during that routine, toys or other objects used, and prompts to elicit child behaviors. Figures 5.3–5.5 provide examples of completed checklists for different children who are described in detail next.

Practitioners should complete this checklist with the family. Engaging families in this process will help them begin to focus on their child's early communication strengths and challenges. Discussing this checklist with the family provides an opportunity to begin to empower the parents to recognize the communication that is already occurring and to help them expand the possibilities for their child. This conversation also provides an opportunity to acknowledge and thank the family for the support they already are providing their child.

The following three scenarios outline three different child profiles to provide examples of how information obtained in the Checklist of Early Communication Behaviors may be used to make decisions about whether TGI is an appropriate strategy for a child or family. For each of the three profiles, a vignette is presented along with a completed Checklist of Early Communication Behaviors to illustrate how the practitioner used the checklist to capture the child's early communication strengths and challenges. First, read the vignettes, and then review the corresponding checklists. An interpretation of each checklist is provided with the vignette.

Child Profile 1, Sophie: Working Toward Triadic Gaze Production

The practitioner observed Sophie to be energetic and very "people focused," smiling happily but vacantly at her mother with no apparent interest in objects or toys. Even when the practitioner held up a toy in front of her, Sophie showed no interest. She was fixed on faces, often leaning in so that a toy did not block her view of the person's face. When the toy was placed in front of her, Sophie still locked onto the practitioner's face. She was "stuck." It was only with intense effort, shaking the toy while refusing to make eye contact with Sophie, that the practitioner could finally draw Sophie's attention to the toy. Once Sophie made the shift from the practitioner's face to the toy, she could also visually follow the toy as it moved across her visual field.

Figure 5.3 presents the Checklist of Early Communication Behaviors completed for Sophie based on this interaction. Sophie is not yet demonstrating many behaviors considered to be foundational for triadic gaze production. She can look at and sustain her gaze on a person, and even on an object with considerable prompting. She is not, however, showing signs of being able to shift between the two. No vocalizations or gestures are present yet in her repertoire. This profile suggests that Sophie would benefit from working on behaviors foundational to triadic gaze production (e.g., working on consistent single focus behaviors, then dual focus behaviors). A child with a profile like Sophie's is a strong candidate for TGI with the focus being on moving toward triadic gaze production.

Checklist of Early Communication Behaviors

Name: *Sophie*

Foundational Behaviors for Triadic Gaze			Source of Information		Notes
			Caregiver Reported	Practitioner Observed	Activity or Routine, Toys or Objects, People Present, Prompts Used
Gaze	Single Focus	Looks and sustains gaze to a **person***	✔	✔	
		Looks and sustains gaze to an **object***	✔	✔	*Needed considerable prompting to look at toy (shaking toy)*
		Follows a moving **object***	✔	✔	*After getting her attention on toy*
	Dual Focus	Looks back and forth between **two objects***		✔	*During playtime on the floor with Mom: focused on one object at a time—not yet looking back and forth.*
		Looks from **object to person OR person to object***		✔	*Can't yet shift from a person to an object—gets "stuck." Will look at the object when provided a prompt—shaking the object.*
	Triadic Focus	Looks **back and forth** between object **AND** person*			
Vocalizations		Produces **early sounds** (fusses, squeals)		✔	*Open vowels only.*
		Produces **consonants, vowels, and consonant–vowel combinations**			
		Produces **word approximations**			
Gestures		**Leans/reaches** for object **OR** person*			
		Shows, points, gives			
		Uses **gestures** meaningfully (waves hi/bye, covers eyes for Peekaboo)			

*NOTE: Be sure to note if the child also uses vocalizations and/or gestures when looking.

Figure 5.3.   Child Profile 1, Sophie: Working toward triadic gaze production.

Checklist of Early Communication Behaviors

Name: *Jack*

Foundational Behaviors for Triadic Gaze			Source of Information		Notes
			Caregiver Reported	Practitioner Observed	Activity or Routine, Toys or Objects, People Present, Prompts Used
Gaze	Single Focus	Looks and sustains gaze to a **person***	✔	✔	
		Looks and sustains gaze to an **object***	✔	✔	*Also leans/reaches for toys*
		Follows a moving **object***	✔	✔	*If focused on toy, will follow its movement*
	Dual Focus	Looks back and forth between **two objects***	✔	✔	
		Looks from **object to person OR person to object***		✔	*In highchair before snack—Dad offers toys on tray. Jack threw toy to floor, then briefly glanced from toy to Dad when Dad made sound effect to go with throwing toy (auditory prompt!).*
	Triadic Focus	Looks **back and forth** between object **AND** person*			
Vocalizations		Produces **early sounds** (fusses, squeals)			
		Produces **consonants, vowels,** and **consonant–vowel combinations**			
		Produces **word approximations**			
Gestures		**Leans/reaches** for object **OR** person*			
		Shows, points, gives			
		Uses **gestures** meaningfully (waves hi/bye, covers eyes for Peekaboo)			

*NOTE: Be sure to note if the child also uses vocalizations and/or gestures when looking.

Figure 5.4. Child Profile 2, Jack: Working on triadic gaze production.

Checklist of Early Communication Behaviors

Name: *Amelia*

Foundational Behaviors for Triadic Gaze			Source of Information		Notes
			Caregiver Reported	Practitioner Observed	Activity or Routine, Toys or Objects, People Present, Prompts Used
Gaze	Single Focus	Looks and sustains gaze to a **person***	✔	✔	*Using all of these single focus behaviors with vocalizations*
		Looks and sustains gaze to an **object***	✔	✔	*Babbling while looking*
		Follows a moving **object***	✔	✔	
	Dual Focus	Looks back and forth between **two objects***			
		Looks from **object to person OR person to object***		✔	*Parents unsure, but observed during play and pointed this out to Mom (Mom agrees).*
	Triadic Focus	Looks **back and forth** between object **AND** person*		✔	*Observed triadic gaze several times during bubble play with Mom. Noted to parents. Both agreed she shifts gaze this way during many activities throughout day.*
Vocalizations		Produces **early sounds** (fusses, squeals)	✔	✔	
		Produces **consonants, vowels,** and **consonant–vowel combinations**	✔	✔	*See notes above re: vocalizations with looking.*
		Produces **word approximations**	✔		*Parents can list 5 word approx. used consistently.*
Gestures		**Leans/reaches** for object **OR** person*	✔	✔	
		Shows, points, gives			*Not yet pointing*
		Uses **gestures** meaningfully (waves hi/bye, covers eyes for Peekaboo)	✔	✔	*Waves arms for "all done," raises arms for "so big," covers face for "Where's Amelia?"*

***NOTE:** Be sure to note if the child also uses vocalizations and/or gestures when looking.

Figure 5.5. Child Profile 3, Amelia: Moving beyond triadic gaze production.

Child Profile 2, Jack: Working on Triadic Gaze Production

Jack's parents described their son as being highly motivated by toys. Jack was persistent in reaching for toys that he wanted. When the practitioner held a toy in front of Jack, he reached and reached—and reached some more—but never looked up at the practitioner. It was clear that Jack did not understand that he could influence the practitioner to give him the toy he wanted. In addition, the practitioner observed that Jack's play repertoire was extremely limited; he often would throw a toy once it was in his grasp. Jack did not yet demonstrate "in-out" play (putting objects into containers and taking them out), nor did he demonstrate any interactive or turn-taking play with his family. However, if the practitioner or Jack's mother or father spoke or made a noise when Jack threw a toy, Jack would briefly glance up at the adult, recognizing the adult's addition to his throwing "game."

Figure 5.4 presents the Checklist of Early Communication Behaviors completed for Jack based on this interaction. This checklist presents a different profile than Sophie's—that of a child with an emerging repertoire of early communication behaviors. Jack is showing some foundational skills on which to directly build toward triadic gaze; he is using gaze to sustain attention to objects and people as well as to track objects through space. He is reaching for toys and other objects but is not as motivated by people. The practitioner notes that Jack is producing minimal to no vocalizations. This profile suggests that Jack is demonstrating some strong foundational gaze behaviors that can be built on through TGI to achieve clearer signals of communication, particularly triadic gaze. One goal for Jack is to help him become an intentional and independent communicator and use communication skills to engage with others. A child with this type of profile would benefit from TGI to build their capacity for intentional and independent communication.

Child Profile 3, Amelia: Moving Beyond Triadic Gaze Production

Amelia sat playing happily with a busy box, with the assistance of her mother, who demonstrated how to push a button, close the box, and push the button again. After several demonstrations, her mother leaned back with the busy box in her hands, just out of Amelia's reach. Her mother asked, "Do you want more?" Amelia looked at the toy and reached for a moment. Then, Amelia vocalized while glancing up at her mother and back to the toy, clearly asking for more by using back-and-forth triadic gaze (toy–mother–toy).

Figure 5.5 presents the Checklist of Early Communication Behaviors completed for Amelia based on this interaction. Amelia has a robust repertoire of early communication behaviors across modalities. She is using gaze, vocalizations, and gestures, and she is combining these behaviors to communicate effectively with her mother during play routines. The practitioner's notes suggest that her parents were unsure about Amelia's use of dual and triadic focus behaviors. However, it is clear that the practitioner observed Amelia produce triadic gaze. When brought to the parents' attention, both parents confirmed that Amelia does indeed shift her gaze back and forth between objects and people many times during her day. Amelia is using her gaze intentionally to communicate her desire to the adult. This profile suggests that Amelia would benefit from early communication intervention that moves her into more symbolic forms of communication, such as treatment that focuses on expanding her repertoire of spoken words and representational gestures.

INDIVIDUALIZED FAMILY SERVICE PLAN DEVELOPMENT

The information obtained from intake, the child evaluation, and the assessment ultimately is used to shape how the team and families plan services. This information is synthesized and used to develop the IFSP. The data obtained from the Checklist of Early Communication Behaviors will help the team, including the family, determine whether TGI should be employed as part of Part C services to support a child's engagement and communication within everyday routines and activities. If TGI is appropriate for a particular child and family, the practitioner should work to incorporate wording that reflects an emphasis on engagement and communication in the IFSP goals. This wording would describe the behavioral achievements that are desired within the context of relevant family routines. Next, sample goals for two of the child profiles, Sophie and Jack, are provided. These IFSP goals focus on using TGI as a strategy for building a child's capacity for social relationships, engagement, and independence. For each IFSP goal, the family's priority is described along with one routine or activity identified by the family that could be used to address this goal. Note that producing triadic gaze is not the first objective for both children. Rather, the most appropriate early communication behavior (gaze, gesture, vocalization) from the continuum is selected as a target behavior for each child based on individual strengths and needs.

IFSP Example: Child Profile 1, Sophie

Recall from Child Profile 1 that social engagement is one of Sophie's strengths, but she can get stuck on faces. Part of the work toward building Sophie's independence and communicative competence will focus on helping her to be able to shift her gaze from a person to an object (e.g., toys) during play routines. For children like Sophie, targeting foundational behaviors along the communication continuum, such as attending to objects (e.g., looking at the ball, reaching), is part of the foundation work needed before targeting more sophisticated behaviors such as triadic gaze.

Family's Priority   Sophie's parents explain, "We want Sophie to play with her older brother and sister. She adores both of them—they make her laugh and smile more than anyone else! But right now, she just watches them having fun; she's not really part of the action. She could just sit and watch them forever. We would love to see her actually participate or take a turn in their games."

Identified Routine and/or Activity   Sophie's siblings spend about 10 minutes playing together in the mornings, right before getting on the school bus. Mom is usually sitting with the children during this time while Dad packs up the kids' lunches. Sometimes the older kids will toss a ball back and forth outside as they wait for the bus to arrive or play with toys inside as they wait.

Possible IFSP Goal   During their morning play routine, Sophie will take a turn playing with toys with her brother and sister by looking at the toy and/or leaning forward to reach for it when one of her siblings holds it up and asks, "Do you want a turn?" three times across 5 days.

IFSP Example: Child Profile 2, Jack

Recall from Child Profile 2 that Jack is highly motivated by toys and focuses on them almost to the exclusion of those around him. When he plays, however, he is not yet acting on objects in a functional way. Most of his play consists of throwing. Jack is just beginning to show that he understands the power of roping in an adult communication partner to help him accomplish a goal, such as getting to a desired toy. Jack will need to learn to shift his attention from toys to adults as a first step in becoming an independent communicator.

Family's Priority   Jack's parents explain: "We want Jack to stop throwing things. We just don't know how to get him to play with toys instead of throwing them. When we bring him something we think he wants, he only holds onto it for a moment and then tosses it aside, but then he gets frustrated because the toy is out of his reach. Instead of asking us for help, he just sits and yells as he looks at the toy across the room. It's so frustrating."

Identified Routine and/or Activity   After Jack's naptime, Jack's dad spends about 15 minutes trying to play with Jack in his room before bringing him to the kitchen for an afternoon snack. Jack has a lot of toys in his room, but Dad has not found one that Jack will play with consistently.

Possible IFSP Goal   During afternoon playtime with his dad, Jack will request a toy that he has thrown out of reach by looking from the toy to his dad and vocalizing five times within 15 minutes of play across 3 days.

CONCLUSION

This chapter provided guidance to assist early intervention practitioners to determine if TGI is a good fit to support families in achieving goals and objectives for their children. The chapter demonstrated how this decision could easily be integrated into commonly used procedures for enrolling a child and family into Part C EI services. Figure 5.6 summarizes this process, including specific information that can be gained during each step for determining the appropriateness of TGI for a family's support services.

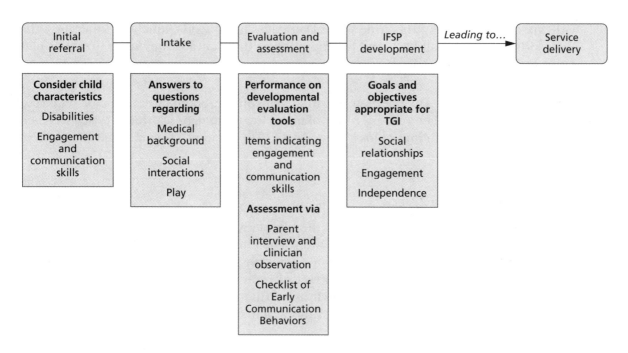

Figure 5.6. The early intervention process and corresponding information for considering appropriateness of Triadic Gaze Intervention. (*Key:* IFSP, individualized family service plan; TGI, Triadic Gaze Intervention.)

As practitioners move forward in the process, they arrive at actual service delivery. Chapter 6 begins to describe in detail how TGI will look when implemented with families. It will walk the reader through PoWRRS-Connect, the six-element protocol for administering TGI. Chapter 7 will follow with suggestions for putting PoWRRS-Connect into action with individual families.

CHAPTER 6

The Essential Elements of PoWRRS-Connect

Delivery Guidelines

TGI is designed to strengthen engagement and communication between families and their children with disabilities. It serves as a strategy for encouraging children's productions of conventional preverbal communication behaviors, consisting of gaze, gestures, and vocalizations, within the context of natural, **authentic routines**. The context for delivering TGI not only encourages successful interactions, but it also highlights experiences that can teach knowledge of objects and object relations, specifically, using the adult as an agent to achieve a desired end goal. TGI should facilitate intentional communication, along with cognitive processes of attending, discovering meaning in actions, generalizing from one experience to another, and determining what actions lead to success.

This chapter describes in detail the six essential elements composing PoWRRS-Connect, the protocol employed in TGI (i.e., provide opportunity, wait, recognize and respond to the child's attempt to communicate, shape to a clearer behavior, and connect). The chapter guides practitioners through the administration of PoWRRS-Connect. The first section of the chapter gives a quick review of the six essential elements and provides an overview of the protocol. Next, the chapter delves into the details for delivering each of the six elements. Opportunities for communication are described first, focusing on choice, requests, and comments. The importance of waiting is then discussed, followed by a close examination of early preverbal behaviors that practitioners and family members should learn to recognize and respond to. Descriptions and video examples are provided to help illustrate each of the behaviors. The element of shaping is then described, exploring the purpose of shaping and actual hands-on procedures. This section of the chapter ends with a description of the last element, connect, which includes a discussion of key features and explores the importance of play with toys as a context for engaging and communicating. **NOTE:** To illustrate how the elements are put together, Appendix C at the end of this book discusses videos of three different children engaged in PoWRRS-Connect and describes the content of each video. These videos are available for streaming at the Brookes Download Hub.

A lot of detail is offered here to facilitate understanding of the essential elements of the intervention protocol. The truth of the matter is that this detail will likely make the protocol feel hard to learn. It might even appear overwhelming. It is not! The chapter is meant as a resource. It provides numerous examples and attempts to reflect the thinking behind these examples. The chapter should be revisited over time to appreciate some of the tips that are given. The heart of the protocol is a very natural connection between adult and child. We hope practitioners and parents will adopt the protocol to fit their styles and meet the needs of the children; this will be done by experimenting, making mistakes, and finding a rhythm.

> *Warning:* Do not get hung up on the details! Make the protocol fit the needs of your child and your style!

TGI: HOW IT LOOKS—MEET PoWRRS-CONNECT

As introduced in Chapter 4, TGI is implemented through a six-element protocol described by the acronym PoWRRS-Connect, which is conceived of as being delivered in a cycle. This cycle is depicted in Figure 6.1: 1) provide opportunity, 3) wait, 4) recognize, 5) respond to the child's communicative attempt, 5) shape, and 6) connect. Another way to think about the implementation of the six elements is to think about the flow of a possible interaction using PoWRRS-Connect. Figure 6.2 provides a diagram illustrating this flow, and **Video 6.1, PoWRRS-Connect Flow**, illustrates it. The video and description that follows is meant as an overview of PoWRRS-Connect and will serve as a template for the elaboration of each element as the chapter unfolds.

The PoWRRS-Connect interaction starts within a natural routine or activity between adult and child (e.g., eating breakfast), where both participants are involved in and attending to each other. The first element requires that the adult pause during the routine and **provide a clear opportunity** for the child to participate or take a turn. In the video, notice the child is having breakfast (yogurt). He is seated in a chair that nicely supports the trunk and head at midline. The adult is sitting directly across from him and at eye level, feeding him one spoonful of yogurt at a time. The first element of the PoWRRS-Connect protocol indicates that the adult provides an opportunity for the child to make a **choice** or a **request**;

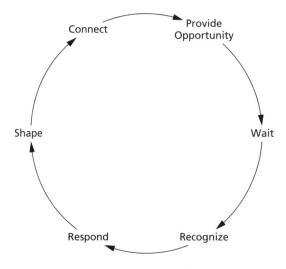

Figure 6.1. PoWRRS-Connect six-element cycle.

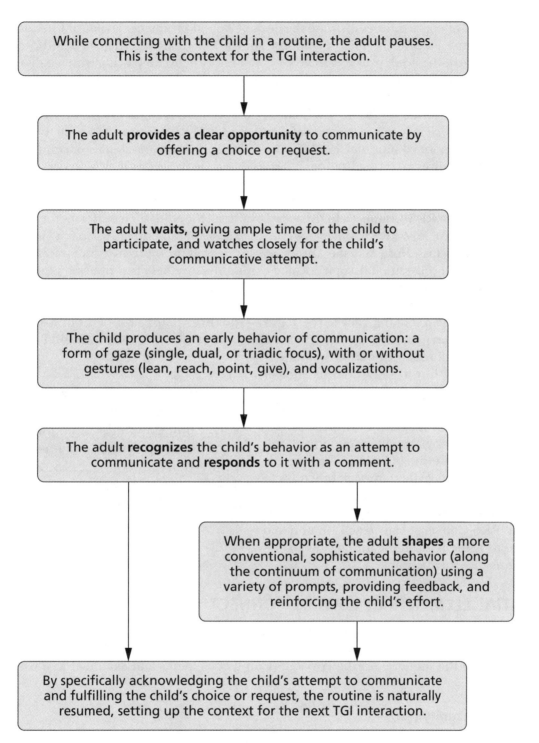

Figure 6.2. PoWRRS-Connect flow. (*Key:* TGI, Triadic Gaze Intervention.)

these types of opportunities increase the odds of a child producing a behavior because these opportunities naturally require a response. In the video, after giving the child two spoonfuls of yogurt, the adult provides a choice opportunity between playing with a ball or taking another bite of yogurt. This is a good choice opportunity because the adult knows the child is enjoying the food but also knows he likes playing with the ball. Notice how she holds the ball up slightly to the side while still holding the spoon on the other side. After the opportunity, the adult clearly *waits* (the second element of PoWRRS-Connect) for the child to produce one or more communication behaviors; these are the early signals of communication (eye gaze, gestures, and vocalizations). Recall that gaze behaviors may be accompanied by a gesture and/or a vocalization. In the video, the child looks at the yogurt and vocalizes. The adult *recognizes* the child's signal and interprets it as the child choosing the yogurt (the third element of PoWRRS-Connect). In this video example, the adult then performs the fourth and fifth elements of PoWRRS-Connect together by *responding* and directly *shaping*. Her response acknowledges his effort, but she knows he can do a little more to communicate. So, she **shapes** a more conventional, sophisticated communicative behavior by asking him to "Look back at your choice." This simple verbal prompt is enough to get the child to look back at the yogurt, which completes the production of a triadic gaze (looking at the yogurt, looking up at the adult, then looking back at the yogurt—the three-point gaze). Part of *responding* and *shaping* includes providing feedback to the child and reinforcing their attempt. In the video, the adult reinforces the child's communication by giving him the yogurt (his choice) and saying, "You got it, buddy. There you go. You told me you wanted more to eat." The last element of PoWRRS-Connect is *connect*, which brings the interaction back full circle to the routine of eating. The choice is offered as part of the routine; it functions to build in a natural communicative exchange with the child. Thus, the six elements of PoWRRS-Connect can teach intentional signals while reinforcing an engaged, communicative interaction.

> *Reminder:* Visit the Brookes Download Hub to access and stream video clips illustrating children's communication behaviors and adults' implementation of the PoWRRS-Connect protocol for Triadic Gaze Intervention. See "About the Video Clips and Downloads" at the front of this book for details about how to access this content.

ESSENTIAL ELEMENTS OF PoWRRS-CONNECT

The six individual elements provide the structure for the flow described. On the surface, these elements seem clear-cut, but each has some intricacies that are worth noting. Tips for addressing the subtleties of the PoWRRS-Connect elements and examples to illustrate are offered next.

Provide Opportunity (Po)

Every cycle starts within the context of an interaction or connection between adult and child. The adult and child should be in close proximity. The child should be alert and demonstrating active interest in their surroundings, particularly the adult. The child should be attending to the adult and the adult attending to the child. *Providing an opportunity* occurs in this context and refers to the adult setting up a clear occasion for the child to engage and communicate with the adult. Worth noting is that not all moments are good for offering an opportunity. If the child is drowsy, is irritable, or just does not seem alert, the adult should pass and try again at another time. The key to success is that PoWRRS-Connect is fun for both the adult and the child. In summary, a clear opportunity consists of the following key features:

- The child is actively attending to the routine or activity with the adult (e.g., looking at the adult or at an object). This can be a familiar or novel routine.

- The routine is interrupted (e.g., the adult pauses in the middle of exploring or manipulating a toy or object, giving a snack, performing an action). Some sense of anticipation occurs in the adult's delivery of the pause, as expressed through facial expression and demeanor.

- The adult provides a verbal cue to elicit participation from the child (e.g., "Which one do you want?" "Do you want more?").

The essence of this element is that it breaks up the flow of an ongoing interaction and provides an obvious chance for the child to communicate. PoWRRS-Connect encourages **choice** and **request opportunities** during social interactions as they are quite salient and provide clear opportunities for a child to communicate and exert control over their world. These two communicative intentions (choosing and requesting) naturally occur in everyday routines, and families should easily grasp how to use them. However, other opportunities, particularly **commenting opportunities**, can provide a way to engage children in other communicative intents. The remainder of this section provides details about choice, request, and commenting, and emphasizes the importance of including each within an engaging routine. *Remember:* Opportunities occur throughout the day and throughout routines. Opportunities to share between adult and child will present themselves in many ways. The guidelines that are provided here highlight how to set them up. Providing opportunities eventually will become second nature to families and mix in naturally throughout the day. Figure 6.3 provides the key features for providing a choice or request opportunity.

Everyone wants a turn to participate; sometimes they need to be invited.
What does a good communication opportunity look like?
1. Actively involve the child in an appealing routine (familiar or novel). Make sure the child is interested and looking at the adult or objects (e.g., play a stacking game with blocks).
2. Interrupt the routine by pausing and showing anticipation for a request (e.g., stop stacking and hold a block up, look at the child and back to the block) or hold up a second toy for a choice (e.g., a ball).
3. Provide a verbal cue to elicit participation from the child; questions work well (e.g., "Do you want more block?" "Do you want the block or the ball?").

Figure 6.3. Key features of providing an opportunity in PoWRRS-Connect.

| **Everyone wants enough time to take a turn in a conversation.** |
| What does good waiting look like? |
| 1. Following the presentation of the elicitation question, pause and wait for approximately 10–15 seconds, or a length of time that is appropriate for the child. *Remember:* Some children need a lot of time to show their best performance, and some need very little time. |
| 2. Stay engaged, looking at the child with anticipation. |
| 3. Wait long enough, but not too long, because the child might lose interest. |

Figure 6.4. Key features of waiting in PoWRRS-Connect.

Choice Opportunities   Choice opportunities include offering the child a choice between two objects or items held before the child in a natural routine (see Figure 6.4). Any two items will work as long as they are interesting to the child and are logical choices for the situation (e.g., two toys, two food items, two clothing items). As the items are being held up for the child, the adult asks a choice question, "Which one do you want, the X or the Y?" (e.g., "Do you want the ball or the bubbles?"). Note that the child should be interested in the items and looking at them.

This may seem simple enough, but there are some subtle aspects to delivering a choice opportunity. Here are some tips to help with administration.

Draw Attention to Two Familiar Items   At the beginning of the opportunity, the child needs to be attending to each item being presented and be familiar with its use or appeal. For example, for a food item, the adult might say, "Do you want the banana or the cracker?" (giving each a little shake to capture the child's looking). "You like bananas, and you like crackers. Which one do you want?" In an ideal situation, the child should look at each item, maybe even scan between them. The adult should encourage this looking by prompting in some way (e.g., shaking items, holding them up, moving items close then apart). Note that some children may fixate on a favorite item and not attend to the second option presented. The adult should try to draw the child's attention to the second item. Once the child has attended to, and possibly scanned between, the two toys and/or food items, the adult should say or repeat, "Do you want the X or the Y?" (naming each item).

Consider Child Preferences   The adult should consider child preferences for toys or food. Sometimes pairing a favorite item with a new item is a good way to stimulate choice. Two favorite items usually work well. Even two new items can be appealing. The adult should think about these variations and try to determine if one works better than another for eliciting the child's interest and participation.

Ask an Elicitation Question   After setting up the choice between items, ask an elicitation question to clearly signal to the child that it is their turn to communicate. For choice opportunities, questions can be general or specific: "Which one do you want?" or "Do you want the X or the Y?"

Present Opportunities Naturally and Repeatedly Choice opportunities can be naturally presented three different times during play with toys and snack.

1. To start an activity or routine, offer a choice such as

   - "Which toy do you want to play with, the ball or the blocks?"

   - "What do you want, juice or cracker?"

2. When making the transition from one toy or snack item to another within an activity or routine, look for opportunities to offer choice. The adult will need to read and interpret the child's cues to see if the child is ready for a choice (e.g., is the child showing restlessness, looking away, or pushing items away?). The adult should verbalize this interpretation with a comment such as

   - "Oh, you don't seem to want to play with that ball anymore."

   - "Oh, you seem to be done with the juice."

   Then, ask the child if they want something else. Once the child has signaled a desire to make a transition, offering a choice between the old item and a new one often should elicit an active response.

3. To provide some variation within the activity or routine, offer choices such as

   - "Do you want the car to go down the ramp or over the bridge?"

   - "Do you want this big monster bite of sandwich or this tiny mouse bite of sandwich?"

Video Examples of Choice Opportunities Videos of two children are provided to illustrate different types of choice opportunities. In the first video **(Video 6.2, Choice, Examples 1–2),** you will see a child in a highchair. This video illustrates two examples of offering a choice. In the first opportunity, at the start of the video, the adult presents a choice between a blue ball and a music box. (*Note:* The child had been playing with the music box prior to the start of the video.) In this opportunity, the adult holds up the two toys at eye level and waits for the child to signal her choice. Notice both the wait time and that the adult is quiet and simply holding the toys up for the child to choose. The child chooses the music, clearly looking back and forth between the music box and the adult, while holding her arms up and vocalizing. This is a nice, clear triadic gaze to say, "I want the music box!" The adult recognizes the communicative behavior and responds to it by winding the music box and presenting it to the child to play. This interaction then makes the transition to the adult offering another choice between two different toys: a red squishy ball and a ring tower. Again, the adult holds up the two toys at eye levels but far enough apart to require the child to look at both toys. After glancing at both toys, the child chooses the ring tower, looking at it and vocalizing excitedly. She tries to reach, looking first at the adult and then back to the toy. She then does another look at the adult and back to the toy. The adult acknowledges her communicative behavior ("You're looking at it") and gives the child the toy.

In the second video, also illustrating a choice opportunity **(Video 6.3, Choice, Example 3),** you will see a child in a highchair playing with her mom. There is a mirror behind the child to allow you to see her mom's actions. The mom offers her child a choice between blocks and beads in a container. Notice that Mom is sitting at midline and eye level and is holding the toys within her child's visual range. The child is definitely engaged; she is actively looking and vocalizing. Mom asks, "Do you want the blocks or the beads?" The child responds by looking at the blocks and vocalizing. She seems to try to reach, but because of her motor impairments (cerebral palsy), she has an extremely difficult time doing so. Mom then waits, holding the toys in position while her child works hard to bring her eyes from her chosen toy back to Mom in midline. During this period, Mom occasionally acknowledges the child's vocalizations and her visual choice by repeating or asking, "You want to play?" At this point in the interaction, it may feel difficult to wait, but watch what happens when Mom continues to wait! The practitioner (off camera to the side) comments, "This is where it's hard for her to get back to you." At that point, the child moves her left arm down, which seems to "release" her to look back at Mom to complete the triadic gaze. Both the practitioner and Mom reinforce her looking; Mom saying, "You found me," and then Mom resumes her play. This beautifully illustrates a successful choice opportunity, along with the waiting that is often necessary for a child to produce a communicative behavior.

Request Opportunities   Request opportunities can include requesting an object out of reach or requesting more of an action that was paused, either using a favorite object or during a fun, social game with the adult. The essence of the request opportunity is that the child needs help and needs to ask for it (e.g., getting help overcoming a barrier or continuing an action). Request opportunities may be less concrete and/or less clear than choice opportunities, but they actually can occur more naturally and frequently throughout most routines.

This may seem simple enough, but there are some subtle aspects of delivering a request opportunity. Here are some tips to help with administration.

Consider Variations and Their Potential Benefits   There are many variations to these types of request opportunities using toys, snack, and activities during social play (e.g., singing songs, playing peekaboo). *Remember:* Toy play has the added benefit in that it builds knowledge of objects and object relations, and concepts of means/ends (i.e., knowledge of agency, someone other than the child acting on an object).

Ensure Child Is Attending and Participating   At the beginning of the opportunity, the child needs to be attending to the item being presented and understand its function or appeal. The adult might need to demonstrate a toy or start a social game to get the child interested, attending, and participating in the routine. The essence of requesting is placing an obstacle in the way of the child or interrupting something ongoing, both of which will elicit a request for help.

Ask an Elicitation Question   An elicitation question should always be asked to clearly signal to the child that it is their turn to communicate. For request opportunities, questions can be general or specific: "Do you want more?" or "Do you want to X again?"

Present Opportunities Naturally and Repeatedly   Request opportunities can be naturally presented in two different ways during play with toys, snack, and social play.

1. Provide an obstacle to start a routine:

    *   The adult can bring out an item behind or in a barrier, such as a tiny toy dog in a clear container. The adult should show the container to the child, shake it, make facial expressions of excitement, and, if appropriate, give the container to the child

and wait as the child examines it. The adult then asks, "Do you want help?" "Do you want the doggy?" or "Do you want me to open it?"

- The adult might show the child a box of juice during snack time and pretend to take a drink, asking the child, "Do you want me to open it?" or "Do you want some juice?"

- The adult might bring out a towel and say to the child, "Do you want to play Peekaboo?"

2. Interrupt a routine by introducing an obstacle:

- The adult can stop any routine or activity with a child and wait to see if the child indicates they want the routine or activity to continue. For example, while rolling a ball back and forth with a child, the adult could stop the activity and ask, "Do you want me to roll the ball to you?"

- During an interruption in an activity, beware; a child may protest if a toy or snack item is removed. In these cases, the adult should make a game of the task. Establishing a turn-taking play routine may be helpful (e.g., "I'll take a turn. Then, you take a turn"); so may playing Hide and Seek, where the adult puts the toy in a container (e.g., "I'm hiding the doll. Can you get her?").

Video Example of a Request Opportunity   To illustrate a **request opportunity**, one video is offered here **(Video 6.4, Request).** In this video, you will see a child in a highchair with the adult demonstrating a busy box toy, playing with it by pushing the separate pieces down, one by one. The child is actively attending and engaged. The adult moves the toy out of the child's reach and asks, "Do you want it again?" and then waits. The child's excitement at requesting triggers some overflow movement (hands raised up and leaning back against the highchair a bit forcefully). The adult repeats, "Do you want it again?" and you will see the child look back and forth between the toy and the adult; this clear triadic gaze, while trying to reach, signals she wants to play with the busy box some more. The video ends with the adult and child connecting and playing.

Commenting Opportunities   Choice and request opportunities have been highlighted as a way to provide a clear opportunity for engaging and communicating because they provide clear indications to a child that it is time for them to participate in the interaction. Choice and request clearly signal that the turn is being passed to the child. This does not mean that an opportunity can only take place in these contexts. Adults can set up other opportunities for a child to communicate. An important one is commenting. Commenting is child initiated and as such is hard to elicit. The communicative interaction is one where the child is motivated to comment on something. The adult can try to facilitate this motivation and elicit a comment, but the requirement for a child to "communicate" is not inherent. Here are some tips for eliciting commenting from a child.

The adult can give the child an opportunity to comment on interesting sights and sounds or on actions. The goal is to take advantage of any situation that might get the child to comment. This is a wonderful, basic part of joint engagement. The adult might do any of the following:

- Present something new, attractive, and interesting, and wait.

- Vary what is being done (i.e., doing something out of the ordinary; for example, in a sing-along game, the adult might start dancing), and wait.

- Make a silly action or sound, look at the child with anticipation, and wait.

- Bring out a wrapped box or decorated bag with something in it. Shake it and wait.

- Follow the child's lead and comment or say something silly about what the child is doing; the child may comment back by looking, gesturing, or vocalizing.

Video Example of a Comment Opportunity   To illustrate a comment opportunity, one video is offered here **(Video 6.5, Comment).** This example demonstrates introducing a surprise toy to a child and waiting for a response. In this video, you will see a child in his wheelchair. The adult plays a chirping bird, which is out of the child's sight. Note his expression stays the same while the bird is chirping, suggesting that he is listening. Once the bird stops, the adult waits with anticipation. This boy, who has severe motor impairments, slowly tries to move his head and trunk to midline so he can look at the adult and smile. This extreme effort to make eye contact, a communicative behavior, clearly signals he is trying to comment on the bird chirping. The adult interprets it that way and reinforces his effort by first acknowledging his behavior as communicative and then by showing him the bird. Watch the child smile as the adult acknowledges his efforts!

Table 6.1 provides additional examples of choice, request, and comment opportunities.

Mixing Choice, Request, and Commenting Opportunities   Although request, choice, and commenting opportunities have been described separately, their delivery can and should be mixed. The opportunities will feel more natural this way. Some key points to remember are as follows:

- Providing communication opportunities gives the child a sense of control in their daily routine, even though the adult is actually maintaining control.

- Many ordinary opportunities will occur throughout the day. Presenting a child two items sets up a choice. Stopping a routine opportunity sets up a request. Offering a unique or surprise object sets up a comment. All kinds of routines offer the context for these opportunities: bath time, play with toys, book reading, bedtime, diaper changing time. The opportunities are meant to be natural and spontaneous. After some practice, they will fit in easily during interactions.

- *Remember:* Playtime with toys adds the extra bonus of stimulating cognitive development. The adult should consider which toys are being selected for playtime; as long as the toys are appealing and appropriate for the child, communication opportunities can easily occur once the child is attending. Think about adaptive toys and how they might be used to stimulate engagement, communication, and play for children with severe motor impairments.

- If the child has had limited experience with play or the child's abilities significantly limit play, be prepared to use hand-over-hand assistance and guidance.

Wait

Following the presentation of an opportunity, the adult needs to wait for the child to produce a communicative behavior (behaviors are described in detail next). The waiting should last approximately 10–15 seconds to give the child enough time to produce the communicative

Table 6.1. Characteristics and examples of good choice, request, and comment opportunities

Characteristics of a good opportunity	Examples	
	Materials	Presentation
Choice		

During any routine with a child, the adult presents two items (two choices) to the child.
 	
The items should be
• Appealing, familiar
• Noticeably different from one another
• Within the child's visual field, including appropriate height
 	
The child should be
• Attending, interested
	Toys: rainstick and ball	At the beginning of a playtime, the adult reaches into a bag and takes out two items. The adult then
		• Holds up, names, and demonstrates each:
		  "Look here's the rainstick. Listen, it makes noise." (Adult turns the stick.) "And here's a ball; it's a bouncy ball." (Adult bounces the ball.)
		• Holds the toys about 10 inches apart, ensures the child has gazed at each one (shaking and renaming as needed), and asks:
		  "Which one do you want?"
		• If necessary, repeats the question and shakes each toy:
		  "Do you want the rainstick or the ball?"

	Snack: toast and banana	In the middle of a snack that includes toast and a banana, where the adult has been alternating between the food items, the adult pauses and
		• Holds up each food item, naming each:
		  "Look, here's your toast and your banana."
		• Tries to hold each item about 10 inches apart, makes sure the child has seen each one.
		• Then asks:
		  "Which one do you want? The toast (as she holds it up) or the banana (holding it forward next)?"

	Getting dressed: two different pairs of socks	The adult is trying to get a child dressed in the morning. Offering choices of clothing can be easy and fun. The adult can
		• Hold up two pairs of socks, describing each one:
		  "Look, here's your favorite blue socks, or maybe you want to try these new green ones."
		• Hold each pair so the child can see each one.
		• Then ask:
		  "Which ones today?"

Request		
During any routine the child is actively participating in, the adult somehow interrupts the flow by stopping or pausing the activity in a way that the child needs help in continuing: • Placing an item out of a child's reach or behind an obstacle. • Operating a toy the child cannot operate on their own • Playing a game that requires an adult take a turn	Toys: bubbles with jar and bubble wand	During playtime with bubbles, several opportunities for request can be offered. The adult • Holds up the bubble wand and demonstrates by blowing bubbles: "Look at this." "Wow, look at all the bubbles." • Stops the activity, and waits, asking, "Do you want more bubbles?" • Continues this, putting the want in and out of the jar, while saying "in" and "out." • Pauses the activity and asks, "Do you want more?" • This kind of activity can have many embedded opportunities: putting the wand in and out and blowing the bubbles.
	Snack: cup of juice	During snack time, the adult • Gives the child a drink of juice. • Holds the juice container just out of the child's reach and asks, "Do you want more?" "Do you need more juice?"

(continued)

Table 6.1.   *(continued)*

Characteristics of a good opportunity	Examples	
	Materials	Presentation
Comment		
Comments are motivated by the speaker and therefore are hard to elicit by others. Setting up an opportunity for a comment works best when something unexpected happens. • Think about an element of surprise, such as an unexpected sight or sound.	Social play: funny face	Face to face with child, the adult • Makes a funny face and sound, then pauses. • Makes another funny face and different sound, then pauses. • Makes a third funny face and a different sound, pausing, saying "silly mommy." • Pausing gives the child an opportunity to react.
	Toys: box of blocks with child's favorite stuffed animal hidden inside	Adult brings out the box of blocks and says, "Let's play with the blocks." Next, the adult • Takes out a block, and says, "Look, one block." • Takes out a second block, says, "Another block" and stacks it. • Takes out a third block, says, "Look, another block" and stacks it. • Then takes out the stuffed animals, and with excitement, says, "Oh, look what I found," pausing, waiting for the child to react.

behavior that comes most easily and naturally to them. Sometimes, waiting a little longer after the child first responds will elicit an even more sophisticated behavior. Triadic gaze paired with gestures and vocalizations is the ultimate set of conventional behaviors the adult wants to see. Look for it, but typically an earlier communicative behavior will likely be produced. Waiting is essential to give the child time to communicate. Each opportunity needs to be clear, as does the wait time. The critical part of waiting is the timing. There is a delicate balance involved in waiting long enough to ensure the child is demonstrating a communicative signal but not so long as to lose the child's interest in the presented activity or toy.

> Waiting is a balancing act: Waiting long enough to ensure the child has time to produce a communicative behavior but not so long as to lose the child's interest.

Ten to fifteen seconds will feel like a long time, but some children will need this much time to respond. This is particularly true for children with motor impairments. In addition, some children may be new to being asked to communicate (i.e., make a choice or request) with their play partner; they, too, may require more time. Other children will find 10–15 seconds intolerably long; they will need a short wait time in order to maintain attention. These might be children who have short attention spans and reduced exposure to play opportunities. Waiting can be a bit tricky; the key is waiting for a behavior that can be recognized and labeled. Consider child characteristics and try to vary wait time to get it just right. See Figure 6.4 for the key features of waiting.

Video Example of Waiting   To illustrate the importance of **waiting**, one video (**Video 6.6, Waiting**) is provided. This video illustrates a boy in his chair playing with an adult who is sitting at eye level in front of him. This video illustrates the importance of waiting, particularly for children with severe motor impairments. This boy has extremely high tone and a strong asymmetrical tonic neck reflex that pulls him away from midline. In this video, the adult presents the child with a choice between a book and a ball spinner. The boy has played with both in the past and liked doing so. The adult sets up a clear opportunity by asking, "The spinner, or shall we do the book?" while she makes sure he has looked at both. The child vocalizes, tries to reach, and makes a tremendous effort to look at the toy he wants, the book. The adult's waiting gives him the extra time he needs to move his head/eyes across midline to gaze in the direction of the book. You will see the adult reinforces his effort by giving him his choice. Video 6.3, which was introduced previously, provides another good example of extended waiting when a child needs that extra amount of time to shift gaze.

Recognize and Respond

Following the presentation of the opportunity and waiting, the child will produce a behavior. The children will likely be new to initiating and maintaining communicative interactions with partners. They will show a variety of behaviors, requiring the adult to be sensitive to what each child brings to the interaction. Recognizing the child's attempt to communicate is critical and oftentimes can be challenging. The adult should pay attention to the child and look for any type of behavior, conventional or unconventional, clear or subtle. Once a communicative attempt is recognized, the adult will then try to interpret the meaning of the communication. Figure 6.5 highlights the key features of recognizing in PoWRRS-Connect.

The real trick to recognizing a child's communicative attempt is identifying what can often be subtle behaviors. A child might produce one or more of the behaviors on the communication continuum, as presented in the Checklist of Early Communication Behaviors, Figure 6.6. (Recall this checklist was introduced in Chapter 5 and used as part of assessment.) Otherwise, the child might produce idiosyncratic behaviors (e.g., moving into a full-body extension to request or maybe showing an overall change in alertness or a slight move of a finger). Recognizing child attempts is critical for establishing engagement and building turn taking. The adult should be attentive to all attempts. The hope though, is

Everyone wants their effort to participate to be recognized.
What does good recognizing look like?
1. Pay attention to what the child is doing, and look for any and all communicative attempts, whether conventional or unconventional. *Remember*: Some behaviors might be unclear, subtle, or fleeting. Pay close attention!
2. Determine if the child is attempting to communicate with a gaze, gesture, or vocal behavior (refer to Figure 6.6).
3. Hypothesize what the child might be meaning, given the opportunity that was provided. *Remember:* The child might be saying no or not interested, or the child may be being unclear.

Figure 6.5. Key features of recognizing in PoWRRS-Connect.

Checklist of Early Communication Behaviors

Name:

Foundational Behaviors for Triadic Gaze			Source of Information		Notes
			Caregiver Reported	Practitioner Observed	Activity or Routine, Toys or Objects, People Present, Prompts Used
Gaze	Single Focus	Looks and sustains gaze to a **person***			
		Looks and sustains gaze to an **object***			
		Follows a moving **object***			
	Dual Focus	Looks back and forth between **two objects***			
		Looks from **object to person OR person to object***			
	Triadic Focus	Looks **back and forth** between object **AND** person*			
Vocalizations		Produces **early sounds** (fusses, squeals)			
		Produces **consonants, vowels, and consonant–vowel combinations**			
		Produces **word approximations**			
Gestures		**Leans/reaches** for object **OR** person*			
		Shows, points, gives			
		Uses **gestures** meaningfully (waves hi/bye, covers eyes for Peekaboo)			

*NOTE: Be sure to note if the child also uses vocalizations and/or gestures when looking.

Figure 6.6.   Checklist of Early Communication Behaviors.

that communicative behaviors can be readable and, if possible, conventional. Early communicative behaviors can include any of the following conventional behaviors:

- *Unengaged behaviors:* lack of response or protest

- *Gaze:* single focus on object or adult, dual focus scanning between two objects or between an object and an adult, or triadic focus with a full three-point gaze shift

- *Gestures:* leaning or reaching; showing, pointing, or giving; using gestures meaningfully

- *Vocalizations:* early sounds; consonants, vowels, or consonant–vowel combinations; and word approximations

- *Combinations of conventional behaviors:* gaze combined with gesture or vocalization; gaze, gesture, and vocalization combined

Examples are described in the sections that follow with corresponding video examples. Note that the video clips are relatively short in length, as are the descriptions, so as to draw the viewer's attention to the specific behavior being illustrated. In all of these videos, pay particular attention to what the child is doing!

Unengaged Behaviors   Unengaged behaviors include both unresponsive, uninterested behaviors and protest behaviors. In both cases, the child is saying, "I'm done" or "I'm not interested." For example,

- *No response:* The child might look away, put their head down, or demonstrate passive looking (gaze that seems uninterested, "off in space").

- *Protest:* The child fusses, cries, pushes a toy or snack or the adult's hand away, and so forth.

Gaze   Gaze can be single, dual, or triadic focus gaze (see Figure 6.6). It involves the child looking at an object or objects, at the adult, or at a combination of these.

Single Focus   Single focus gaze means the child looks at an object or at the adult. Single focus gaze is characterized by the following:

- Duration. The child looks at the object or adult (for approximately 3 seconds); if the adult or object moves, the child will follow or track the movement (tracking).

- A sense of persistence in the looking. *Note:* This is very different from passive looking (looking around) or protest. The child is actively focusing on the object or adult in an engaged manner.

- Indication of excitement in body movement or change in facial expression

Video Examples of Single Focus Gaze   Two video exemplars (Videos 6.7 and 6.8) are provided to illustrate single focus. Both occur in choice opportunities. In these short videos, pay particular attention to the child's behaviors.

In **Video 6.7, Single Focus, Example 1**, two toys are presented as a choice: a yellow pom pom and pink tube. Child behaviors to observe are the child looks at and reaches toward the yellow pom pom.

Likewise, in **Video 6.8, Single Focus, Example 2**, two toys are presented as a choice: ball and beads. Child behaviors to observe are the child looks at and reaches for beads while producing a vocalization.

Dual Focus   Dual focus gaze means the child looks between two objects or between an object and person. Typically scanning between objects emerges first. Tracking a single object often can lead to looking between objects.

Dual Focus (Scanning Objects)   With this type of dual focus gaze, the child looks back and forth between two objects. The adult does not get acknowledged by the child, particularly as a possible agent of an action. The look can be quick or quite slow and deliberate.

Dual Focus (Scanning Adult and Object)   With this type of dual focus gaze, the child looks between the object and adult, often after looking between objects. Note that this behavior does not complete the three-point gaze shift (object–adult–object or adult–object–adult). When accompanied by gestures and vocalizations, it can be a strong communicative signal because the child acknowledges both the object and the adult as part of the interaction.

Video Examples of Dual Focus Gaze   Two video exemplars are provided to illustrate dual focus. In both examples, the child looks between objects during choice opportunities (dual focus scanning objects). In addition, in both examples, the child also includes the adult in the scan (dual focus scanning adult and object). In these videos, pay particular attention to the child's behaviors.

In **Video 6.9, Dual Focus, Example 1,** two toys are presented as a choice: slinky and bubbles. Child behaviors to observe are the child looks away, looks at the clinician's face, and quickly scans from the clinician to the bubbles. *Note:* This gaze shift is subtle.

In **Video 6.10, Dual Focus, Example 2,** two toys are presented as a choice: tambourine and slinky. Child behaviors to observe are the child looks at the clinician during the elicitation question, then scans from the tambourine to the slinky (dual focus between two toys). Note that the adult waits a little longer trying to get the most sophisticated signal from the child. The child then looks at the slinky, reaches, and vocalizes before looking down and away. Finally, the child looks at and reaches for the slinky again, and shifts her gaze up to the adult, thus demonstrating a scan object–adult gaze behavior. The adult's waiting allows the child to show her best communicative behavior.

Triadic Focus   In triadic focus gaze, the child completes the three-point gaze shift. Triadic focus gaze has these characteristics:

- The child looks at the object, then at the adult, and finally back at the object—or in the reverse order: adult–object–adult.

- The child appears to acknowledge the role of the adult in the interaction (i.e., the adult serving as the agent of an action).

- The gaze shift should occur within an approximately 5-second time frame to show their link; sometimes, though, the gaze shift is faster.

Video Examples of Triadic Focus Gaze   Two video exemplars are provided to illustrate triadic focus: one during a request opportunity and one during a choice opportunity. Again, in these videos, pay particular attention to the child's behaviors:

Video 6.11, Triadic Focus, Example 1, is the same video clip presented earlier in Video 6.4, but this time, as you watch, focus on the child's behavior. One toy, a busy box, is presented in a request opportunity. After the adult says, "Do you want it again?" the child looks back and forth between the toy and the adult. She exhibits some overflow movement, then again looks back and forth between the toy and the adult, using triadic gaze plus vocalization to request more.

In **Video 6.12, Triadic Focus, Example 2,** two toys are presented in a choice opportunity: a blue ball and yellow pom pom. Significant behaviors are that the child looks at the clinician, scans between the two objects (dual focus), and then shifts his gaze from the blue ball, to the adult, and back to the blue ball with a reach toward the blue ball at the end (triadic focus plus reaching gesture). Note the adult's waiting gives the child enough time to produce the full triadic gaze, which is a clear signal to choose the ball.

As illustrated in the previous video exemplars, gaze can be accompanied by gestures and vocalizations.

Gestures   Gestures include leaning or reaching gestures; showing, pointing, or giving gestures; and meaningful use of gestures (see Figure 6.6).

Leaning or Reaching   Leaning or reaching gestures are characterized by the following:

* The child leans forward in the direction of the object.

* Arms may be up but remain bent, or arms and hands may move in the direction of the object.

* The gesture is always accompanied by sustained looking at the object (i.e., single focus toward the object).

Showing, Pointing, or Giving   Examples of showing, pointing, and giving gestures include the following:

* The child picks up an object or snack and holds it up toward the adult.

* The child extends a finger toward an object.

* The child places an object or snack in the adult's hand.

Using Gestures Meaningfully   Examples of using gestures meaningful are the child waves bye-bye and the child shakes their head "no."

Vocalizing   Vocalizations (see Figure 6.6) can be characterized as follows:

* The child produces early sounds (fussing, squeals).

* The child produces early consonants, vowels, or consonant–vowel combinations: vowel–consonant (VC) combinations, or canonical babbles (CVCV).

* The child produces word approximations (*da* for "that," *mo* for "more").

Eye gaze, gestures, and vocalizations (or even words or signs) may occur alone or in combination, as follows:

* Gaze alone

* Gaze + gesture/or vocalization

* Gaze + gesture + vocalization

Remember: **Recognize** means the adult should look for any and all communicative attempts produced by the child, whether conventional or unconventional. **Respond** means

Everyone wants their effort to participate to be acknowledged.
What does good responding look like?
1. Responding is dependent on recognizing the child's attempt and hypothesizing about what it meant.
2. Name the child's behavior (e.g., "You're looking at the ball") and say its presumed meaning (e.g., "I bet you want it"). Even if in doubt, give it a try (e.g., "I think you are telling me . . .").
3. Act on the meaning (e.g., give the child the ball). *Remember:* These children may be working hard. Show the child that their effort paid off.
4. In natural interactions, sometimes it is difficult or inconvenient to respond immediately, so at least acknowledge the communication (e.g., "I know you want it now, but wait 1 minute while I open the jar").

Figure 6.7.   Key features of responding in PoWRRS-Connect.

the adult should label what the child is doing and how it is being interpreted. The adult should be explicit (e.g., "You're looking at the ball; you're telling me you want it," "You're trying to reach the juice. You want more, don't you?"). It's important to clearly acknowledge the child's effort. Figure 6.7 highlights the key features of responding in PoWRRS-Connect. If the child has put a lot of effort into their attempt, it is fine to recognize, respond, and move on to connect (skipping shaping). This is an important judgment call that is discussed in the next section.

Shape

Shaping is the next element, and it builds from the child's communicative attempt. Think about shaping as praising the child for their effort to communicate and offering a new option for them to try. Shaping assumes that the child's first attempt could be more conventional or sophisticated, and the adult serves as a guide for the child to try a new, clearer behavior. It also assumes that the child is still attending and showing a willingness to try something new. Shaping (also called scaffolding) means helping the child successfully perform a behavior or task that is just beyond their capacity. This is accomplished by structuring the context so that the child can gradually move from performing where the child is comfortable to successfully performing a new, challenging behavior or task. The tricky part is appreciating the child's state and willingness to try again. Shaping every behavior to one that is more conventional or sophisticated can become frustrating for the child and the adult. We advise against that! Focus on maintaining the child's engagement in the interaction and supporting their production of more sophisticated behaviors when it seems right. Figure 6.8 provides the key features of shaping in PoWRRS-Connect.

Shaping Goals   When approaching shaping, the adult needs to assess whether the child could be prompted to produce a more conventional, sophisticated response. This includes

> # Everyone wants to learn.
>
> What does good shaping look like?
>
> 1. Shaping means trying to help the child produce a new, desired behavior using helpful prompts.
>
> 2. Shaping requires the child's attention and interest and should only be done if the child's first behavior was insufficient in some way and the adult believes the child could produce a more readable or conventional behavior. Always be encouraging, and only shape when it feels right!
>
> 3. Consider the materials, and decide how they might be changed to help elicit a new behavior. In a choice opportunity, maybe the child did not see the two items well. Or in a request, maybe the child was not interested. Vary the materials if needed.
>
> 4. Consider the prompts that could be used to help elicit a new behavior (see Table 6.2):
>   - Verbal
>   - Visual
>   - Auditory
>   - Tactile
>
> 5. Offer a prompt, or more than one, to help shape the new behavior. Most prompts are given in combination. Always consider the child's preferences in prompt type and tolerance for trying something new. Try to vary prompts.
>
> 6. Use simple, clear verbal directions to describe what you want the child to do and what the child is doing. Give a lot of praise.
>
> 7. Be creative, and have fun!

Figure 6.8.   Key features of shaping in PoWRRS-Connect.

identifying which communicative behaviors the child typically produces and which prompts or cues might successfully shape the child's performance toward a more sophisticated behavior. Sometimes a single prompt elicits a more sophisticated response. Sometimes a combination of one or more of the four types of prompts—verbal, visual, auditory, and tactile—listed next works best. For example,

- Verbal prompts provide spoken, linguistic input to the child, such as telling the child, "Look at me."

- Visual prompts include moving a toy and/or the adult's face into the child's line of regard.

- Auditory prompts include any nonlinguistic attention-getter, such as activating a musical toy, whistling, or humming.

- Tactile prompts include physically interacting with the child in some manner, such as touching, tapping, or jostling to alert or arouse the child, or providing hand-over-hand assistance with toy manipulation.

Table 6.2 provides definitions and examples of the different prompts used in shaping.

Shaping Procedures   We encourage the adult to tailor shaping procedures to match each child's responsiveness using a variety of these prompts. *Remember:* Four types are available. Try them all during the first several presentations. Be systematic, yet flexible, matching what type of prompt will likely help the child. Do not worry as much about the product, but rather, focus on and enjoy the process. Several videos are provided to illustrate shaping. As you read about shaping and watch the videos, note the variety of techniques that are used. Shaping truly is an art, so be creative in your approach. When trying to shape a more conventional, sophisticated behavior, be mindful of the following:

- What are the child's sensory likes or dislikes (e.g., Do auditory prompts frighten the child? Is the child sensitive to touch?)?

- Which type of prompt will be most useful in obtaining the result you want (e.g., will a verbal prompt get the child's attention to look at you? Will shaking a toy get the child to look back at the toy?)?

Table 6.2. Shaping prompts and examples

Shaping prompts		
Modality	Definition	Example
Verbal	Spoken, linguistic prompts used to shape the child's behavior	Call the child by name. Label the toy(s) presented. Directly prompt the child to perform an action.
Visual	Prompts that involve movement within the child's visual space	Shake, wave, tap, etc., a toy within the child's field of vision. Move a toy or the adult's face into the child's line of vision. Point to a toy and/or the adult's eye(s).
Auditory	Audible but nonlinguistic sounds	Produce nonspeech sounds (e.g., whistles, clicks, finger snapping). Activate a musical component of a toy.
Tactile	Physical interaction with the child	Touch the child's face to gain attention. Place a toy on the child's arm or in the child's hand. Guide the child's hand toward a toy.

- What are adult preferences versus child preferences (e.g., verbal prompts might be most natural, but they may be meaningless or challenging to the child who prefers visual attention-getters or has a difficult time processing spoken input)?

Shaping starts once the child has produced a communicative attempt and the adult believes it is appropriate to shape the next behavior along the continuum. For example, a child produces a sustained single focus or gaze to show engagement with a toy and/or adult. The adult would try to elicit dual focus from the child by doing the following:

- As the child is looking at an object, the adult tries to get the child to shift their look to the adult.

- If the child is looking at one toy when given a choice, the adult tries to get the child to look at the other one, and back and forth between toys.

To give another example, a child produces dual focus and the adult tries to shape triadic focus. In this example, the adult wants to emphasize looking back and forth between object and adult to build the child's connection between the two. This hypothetically might look like the following:

- Shake the toy (visual and auditory prompt); make sure the child is looking at it.

- Then, facilitate spontaneous eye contact—elicit eye movements that signal a connection between the toy and you by doing the following:

  o Gradually moving the toy near your face—with or without shaking the toy (visual prompt) OR

  o Moving your head down to the toy (visual prompt)

- Make a face, make noises (auditory prompt), or otherwise attract the child's attention to you.

- Then, shake the toy again; get the child to look at it.

- Use a variety of prompts to get the child engaged and looking.

- *Remember*: Some children with motor problems have difficulty moving their eyes. Help the child along by moving the toys slowly and waiting.

Video Example of Shaping Dual Focus in a Request Opportunity   **Video 6.13, Shaping, Example 1,** illustrates shaping in a request opportunity. The adult attempts to help the child look from an interesting toy (squishy ball) up to her eyes. The adult specifically is trying to shape single focus (looking at the ball) to dual focus (looking from the ball to her). What you'll see and hear the adult do:

- The adult presents a toy in a request opportunity: squishy ball.

- She says, "Here we go . . . ." (VERBAL)

- She makes sounds, "*Di-di-di-di.*" (AUDITORY)

- She moves the ball toward her face and then shakes the toy. (VISUAL)

When shaping behavior, keep two guidelines in mind:

1. Build on behaviors already present in the child's repertoire.

2. Use simple, direct verbal input to tell the child what you want, describe what the child has done, and verbalize the "signal."

Build on Behaviors Already Present   For children who tend to focus only on objects or only on people, utilize visual tracking as a form of prompt.

- For the child who is focused on the toy, use visual tracking to move the child's eyes toward your face.

- For the child who mostly focuses on people rather than toys, work first on facilitating focus on the toys and play. *Then*, work toward dual and triadic gaze by having the child track the object toward your face.

Video Example of Shaping Triadic Gaze by Building on Existing Behaviors   In **Video 6.14, Shaping, Example 2,** the adult attempts to shape triadic gaze during a request opportunity. She uses a variety of verbal and visual cues to help the child look from a spinner toy, up to her eyes, and back to the spinner toy. What you will see and hear the adult do (although the description below is written sequentially, the prompts overlap in their delivery):

- The adult presents a toy in a request opportunity: spinner ball

- She says, "Should we do more? What do you think? Oh, good reach! Look at me!" (VERBAL)

- She shakes toy in space as it moves. (VISUAL)

- She points to her own eyes. (VISUAL)

- She says, "Look at me." (VERBAL)

- She shakes the toy in space. (VISUAL)

- She says, "Look back at the ball." (VERBAL)

- She ends by saying, "You did it!"

Use Simple, Direct Verbal Input   Use simple, direct verbal input to tell the child what you want, describe what the child has done, and verbalize the "signal." Gauge verbalizations based on the child's cognitive and/or processing level. Some examples include

- "Now look at me!"

- "Find my eyes."

- "You looked at me! You told me you wanted that toy."

- "You are looking at me and the X. You are telling me you want the X." (This helps the child appreciate that triadic gaze is an intentional communicative signal.)

In a choice opportunity, hold up two objects. If the child first looks at each toy, then sustains gaze on one, say, "Oh, do you want this one?"

- Say, "Look at me." (Hold the toy near your face.)

- Shake the toy to get the child to look back at it.

- Verbalize, "You looked at the toy and you looked at me. You told me you wanted more."

Finally, note that verbal prompts are rarely used on their own. Instead, they are often combined with visual, auditory, and/or tactile prompts. Also, beware that there is a tendency to "over-use" verbal prompts, even though other cues may be more salient to children.

Video Example of Shaping Dual Focus in a Choice Opportunity   In **Video 6.15, Shaping, Example 3,** the adult is trying to shape a dual focus between a toy and the adult. This is a choice opportunity, where the adult presents a red truck and a ball. Note how the adult makes sure the child has seen both toys. The child is clearly focused on the truck, and the adult wants to get herself into the interaction with the child. She uses a variety of cues to draw the child's attention and gaze from the truck to the adult. What you will see and hear the adult do:

- The adult presents two toys in a choice opportunity: red truck and blue ball.

- She says, "Do you want the red truck? Marley, look up at me." (VERBAL)

- She tries to guide the child to look up by using her finger and saying, "Find my eyes, Marley." (VISUAL and VERBAL)

- She moves the truck close to her eyes and points to her eyes, saying, "Up here."

- When she makes eye contact with the child, she says, "I see you now" and gives her the truck. This is a clear response to the child's gaze shift.

Video Example of Shaping Gaze and Tracking   In **Video 6.16, Shaping, Example 4,** the adult (an SLP) is working to see if this child can track objects. The child has cerebral palsy with severe motor impairments. The SLP and the mom are working together to shape gaze toward an object and tracking the object. The SLP holds the child on her lap, securing his back and head, while the mother offers two toys, a bouncy toy and a ring ball. What you will see and hear the adults do:

- They present two toys in the choice: bouncy toy and ring ball.

- The SLP instructs Mom to hold up the two toys to see if the child will look between them.

- Mom holds the toys up so he can see them. She then says, "Look here, different. Very different," first letting him feel each toy and then, shaking them. (VERBAL, TACTILE, and VISUAL)

- You might see the child produce a quick gaze shift between the toys.

- To shape tracking, the mom beautifully moves the bouncy toy within the boy's range of vision. (VISUAL)

- The SLP says, "Nice looking; you're looking with your eyes!"

Note this shaping involves both securing the child's positioning (the SLP) and offering toys in a way that the child can see them and with help touch them (Mom). The SLP offers a nice, clear response at the end, describing and reinforcing what the child is doing with his eyes.

Most important, shaping uses a creative assortment of visual prompts, verbal instructions, and tactile cues to actively assist the child in moving from where they are currently functioning to a new level: one that connects people and objects or actions. Eliciting gaze-shift behaviors in this way helps the child see how the adult can be a means to an end. Imagination and judgment are an important part of shaping: use a variety of cues that are appropriate to the child. *Remember:* The goal is to have fun, working with the child in a give-and-take way to encourage new ways to communicate.

Connect

Every communication opportunity ends by supporting the child's communication attempt and engaging/connecting with the child. After all, this engagement/connection is the goal of the communication. The purpose of the previous five elements of PoWRRS-Connect is to ultimately have the child participate in the natural context (i.e., everyday activities and routines, e.g., playtime, snack time, mealtime, bath time). The PoWRRS-Connect cycle ends (and begins) with the routine and the natural interaction. Through the TGI strategy, the child learns they can communicate and be an active, engaged participant in the turn-taking dance with the adult. This connection may include objects or toys.

Playtime with toys is particularly appealing for children with moderate to severe disabilities, particularly motor impairments, as they are often limited in their exposure to toys. Play can be ideal for not only building communication skills but also offering occasions for exploring objects, thus giving children experiences they might otherwise not be getting. Play with toys offers exposure to important concepts of object awareness and object relations, including location relations (e.g., in/on/under), possessive relations (e.g., doll's hat), or means/ends relationships (e.g., adult opening a box). Simply put, playtime offers a powerful context for engaging and communicating.

The connection that follows each opportunity also provides the context for setting up the next opportunity to communicate. This is particularly true for the opportunity types of choice, request, and commenting. The PoWRRS-Connect cycle can be repeated over and over throughout the day in a variety of routines and activities; ideas for doing so are provided in Chapter 8. Figure 6.9 provides a summary of the key features for connecting, and two videos illustrate the importance of connecting through play.

Video Examples of Connecting During Play   The two videos that follow are provided to illustrate the value of play as a way of connecting between adult and child. In these videos, an adult and a child with cerebral palsy and severe motor impairments are interacting. Because of the child's motor involvement, he has difficulty manipulating toys. The beauty

---

Everyone wants the engagement or conversation to continue.
What does good connecting look like?
1. *Remember:* PoWRRS-Connect is a cycle, starting and ending with connecting with the child.
2. Resume the routine and the natural interaction. A routine was interrupted by a clear, salient opportunity to engage or communicate, followed by waiting, recognizing, responding, and shaping, so now it is time to get back to the activity. Continue the routine or move it along.
3. Never make the PoWRRS-Connect protocol too intrusive. It should be natural. Within any routine or activity, look for ways to introduce the protocol in the natural flow of engaging.

Figure 6.9.   Key features of connecting in PoWRRS-Connect.

of these video examples is the way the adult brings him into the play activity by setting up a clear, predictable routine with the toy and calling him by his name. The joy they each experience is a huge part of building new skills through PoWRRS-Connect.

In **Video 6.17, Connect, Example 1,** the adult is playing Peekaboo with a puppy. Note how the adult and child are equally participating, enjoying the moment. The boy's laughter and his gaze to the puppy signal his excitement about the game. This play could naturally lead to a request opportunity, where the adult stops the Peekaboo game and asks the child if he wants more.

Video 6.18, Connect, Example 2, shows the adult demonstrating play with a stacking ring toy. Because of his motor impairments, this child likely has not had many opportunities to explore objects independently or engage in these early play routines without support. The adult uses the toy to engage him but also uses the rings to focus his attention on gaze. To get him more actively involved, she helps him play by moving his arms to bat the toy. She has clearly gotten him engaged with that toy and could naturally set up a choice opportunity between the stacking ring toy and a different toy. In this way, the play can lead to a new communication opportunity.

PUTTING IT ALL TOGETHER

Three additional video examples that illustrate the PoWRRS-Connect cycle are provided in Appendix C. Each video demonstrates how the elements flow together. Descriptions accompany each video that include background information for the children and information about important features of delivery. These videos will help practitioners appreciate how the six elements of PoWRRS-Connect flow together in an easily administered protocol. These videos can also be shown to families to illustrate how PoWRRS-Connect can be easily implemented.

STICK TO THE SIX!

The TGI strategy is structured around the PoWRRS-Connect protocol consisting of six elements described in this chapter. These six elements and the structure should seem straightforward and familiar, as they reflect typical turn taking during communication. What makes the TGI structure different from a typical interaction is that PoWRRS-Connect breaks down and emphasizes the basic, essential parts of turn taking. The PoWRRS-Connect elements describe this turn taking in slow motion. Based on the evidence, if the six elements are implemented as described, the desired outcomes of enhanced engagement and communication between adult and child should follow. The structure is meant as a template for implementing the protocol during various routines and activities in the children's lives. The idea of a template is important. Practitioners and families should be familiar with the six elements and make them their own as they are implemented throughout the day. The consistency and repetition of PoWRRS-Connect during everyday routines allows for building and practicing successful engagement and communication naturally. The beauty of the six-element structure is that families can vary quite a few aspects of delivery, while maintaining its integrity. The variations can include changing materials (i.e., recognizing child preferences), presentation style (i.e., what is said and done), and density of use in any activity (i.e., how often PoWRRS-Connect is used). The expectation is that the six elements will become second nature and families will find ways to use them spontaneously and effortlessly. Sticking with the six elements will form the foundation for ongoing teaching and learning. Sticking to the six elements will better ensure success for building strong communication between children and others. We urge practitioners to return to this chapter as they become more familiar with the protocol and as they instruct families. Families should experiment and not worry about making mistakes; that is how it will become second nature to them.

CONCLUSION

This chapter has provided considerable detail about PoWRRS-Connect. We hope the chapter will serve as an ongoing resource for practitioners as they learn the administration of the protocol. The six essential elements should become second nature to practitioners and ultimately caregivers. Chapter 7 follows with information about how to put PoWRRS-Connect into action with children and their families, including things to consider before implementing PoWRRS-Connect and what a first visit using PoWRRS-Connect might look like.

CHAPTER **7**

Putting PoWRRS-Connect Into Action With Families

This chapter focuses on clinical ideas and techniques that have been identified over the years as valuable for successfully implementing PoWRRS-Connect. Some of the material—maybe all—will seem familiar to practitioners. The information presented here parallels birth-to-three practice and good clinical decision making routinely used by practitioners. Practitioners ideally will read this chapter, recognize and interpret the information from their clinical perspective and experience, and apply it as they work with families learning to use PoWRRS-Connect. The chapter suggests how to incorporate the PoWRRS-Connect ideas and techniques into practice, but ultimately practitioners will do what they do best: work with families.

The chapter is organized into two parts. Part 1 outlines important considerations to review before implementing PoWRRS-Connect, beginning with a discussion about obtaining family buy-in for TGI and using PoWRRS-Connect to accomplish IFSP goals. Next, the chapter discusses family and child characteristics that can influence successful implementation of PoWRRS-Connect. This includes important information about positioning children with motor impairments and identifying which communication behaviors to emphasize in the administration of PoWRRS-Connect for individual children. Part 2 of the chapter takes the reader step by step through the first visit with a family, describing in detail how to use PoWRRS-Connect to address the family's IFSP goals, with examples provided.

PART 1: CONSIDERATIONS BEFORE IMPLEMENTING PoWRRS-CONNECT

Family Buy-In

The first area that practitioners will need to consider before introducing TGI and PoWRRS-Connect to families is buy-in. Every practitioner understands that families must believe in the intervention plan and see themselves as partners with the birth-to-three team in implementing that plan. Therefore, families will need to appreciate the value of TGI and the PoWRRS-Connect protocol and believe that it can easily become part of their everyday routines. Chapters 1 and 2 provide the background on which TGI was created. This background information reviews the value of engagement and preverbal communication as the foundation for later social, cognitive, and language learning, and it provides a strong rationale for explaining the value of TGI to caregivers. The idea of focusing on engagement and communication will be new for many families. They may have other ideas in mind for the services they need. If TGI seems appropriate for a child and family, practitioners will need to offer clear information to encourage the family's consideration of this focus. Families will need to understand the significance of preverbal communication development prior to first words, signs, or symbols. To help caregivers appreciate the importance of engagement and communication during the first year of life, and how to facilitate such development, two caregiver handouts are provided in Appendix D of this book; they are also available on the Brookes Download Hub with the other downloadable resources. The first of these handouts, Early Communication, describes early preverbal development during the first year of life prior to first words, plus it presents the continuum of specific early gaze, gestural, and vocal behaviors that emerge during this time period. Practitioners may wish to share this information with families to explain the importance of early engagement and communication and encourage buy-in for TGI and implementing the PoWRRS-Connect protocol as part of their early support services. The second handout, discussed later in this chapter, guides caregivers through the elements of the PoWRRS-Connect protocol.

> *Reminder:* Consider the following when planning the implementation of PoWRRS-Connect:
>
> Family buy-in to TGI and adopting the protocol
>
> Family characteristics
> - Natural environment
> - Style and preferences
>
> Child characteristics
> - States for engagement
> - Positioning needs
> - Style and preferences
>
> Communication skills and abilities
> - Actual versus potential level of performance

Simply put, TGI offers a chance to improve engagement and communication between children and others. Through the implementation of PoWRRS-Connect, children will learn to produce clearer, more conventional communication behaviors and build successful interactions with others; families will be empowered to support their children's future learning across developmental domains. The PoWRRS-Connect protocol, described in detail in Chapter 6, should be easy to use during natural routines that occur throughout the day, every day. Implementing PoWRRS-Connect should become a regular part of interactions between caregivers and children during play, mealtime, bath time, and any time they are together. Practitioners need to impress on caregivers that the PoWRRS-Connect protocol can help their children become clearer communicators and, in turn, build more successful interactions. Practitioners will need to explain and demonstrate how PoWRRS-Connect is useful for achieving a family's IFSP goals. Families' endorsement of practitioners' suggestions is essential for success. The significance of focusing on engagement and communication—and the value of PoWRRS-Connect and the ease with which it can be delivered—need to be understood and appreciated by families as they partner with practitioners. Figure 7.1 highlights appealing qualities of TGI and the PoWRRS-Connect protocol that practitioners should share with families to encourage buy-in.

Family Characteristics

Using PoWRRS-Connect with families requires understanding and appreciating a family's natural environment as well as their interaction style and preferences. These characteristics, which will vary across (and sometimes within) families, are discussed next.

Family Buy-In: Selling Points for Triadic Gaze Intervention (TGI) and the PoWRRS-Connect Protocol

The TGI strategy emphasizes
- The importance of engaging and communicating, building connections, and interacting with others during the first year of life (a lot happens before first words).

The PoWRRS-Connect protocol is
- A way of helping children produce clearer communication behaviors, particularly gaze, gestures, and vocalizations that
  - Will build successful interactions with others
  - Will enhance future learning across developmental domains
- An easily learned set of six essential elements that
  - Provide a natural way to interact with their children
  - Fit the families' priorities and activities in day-to-day living
- A way of reaching one or more individualized family service plan goals

---

Figure 7.1. Family buy-in: Appealing qualities of Triadic Gaze Intervention and PoWRRS-Connect.

Natural Environment   Families already will have described their routines during the initial assessment (see Chapter 5), but the first visit with the family presents the opportunity to take a deeper dive into this information. The practitioner will want to know which routines families describe as relatively fun and easy versus stressful and hard. A quick reminder: Routines are not just what happens at home but include going out for an activity, such as visiting friends or family, going to child care, shopping, and so forth. Family routines provide the context for planning how to address the IFSP goals. Many IFSP goals center around supporting the child's independence, communication, and social engagement within and across the family's authentic everyday routines and activities. Thus, PoWRRS-Connect can be a truly useful technique to offer families. When the family is just beginning to learn the PoWRRS-Connect protocol, the fun and easy routines might be the focus. This will give both caregivers and children the chance to become familiar with PoWRRS-Connect and allow them to practice and build familiarity and confidence with the six elements. Of course, the PoWRRS-Connect elements are really meant to give caregivers a way of working through the more stressful and difficult routines. More fully integrating the PoWRRS-Connect protocol into challenging routines will need some practice; ideas for helping families in these contexts are described in the second part of this chapter.

Style and Preferences   Family styles and preferences also will need to be considered when supporting families in the implementation of PoWRRS-Connect. As with any part of service delivery, a family's beliefs, values, and cultural practices should be considered in

Table 7.1. Family style and preferences

Style

- Active versus passive

- Talkative versus quiet

- Questioning versus observant

- Directive versus following child's lead

Preferences

- Types of activities and activity locations

- Types of toys

- Times of day

relationship to the strategies that are being suggested. Culture will inherently overlap with style and preferences; sensitivity to and respect for different cultural practices must become part of planning birth-to-three support services and instruction for PoWRRS-Connect. Table 7.1 presents a brief list of family styles and preferences to consider before implementing the PoWRRS-Connect protocol.

Style refers to caregiver personality traits such as level of expressiveness or openness in how they interact with others. Some may be talkative, whereas others are quiet. Some may gesture a lot, whereas others gesture very little. Some may ask others, including their children, a lot of questions, whereas others will sit back and observe or describe. One style is not better than another. Each is worth considering when guiding families in the use of PoWRRS-Connect. Some caregivers may be more direct in how they interact with their children, and this can be a plus in offering choice and request opportunities during PoWRRS-Connect. This style might also make shaping more natural in that the caregiver will be helping the child produce a new communicative behavior. A caregiver who is more direct will need to be cautious about considering the child's attention and interest; however, being direct has the advantage of introducing new toys, ideas, and routines. On the other hand, caregivers that tend more frequently to follow their child's lead may find connecting with their child easier. Following a child's lead almost guarantees having the child's interest and attention. The child's preferences can dominate, which helps show the child they have some control. Following a child's lead can make opportunities for commenting easier in PoWRRS-Connect. As the adult comments on objects and activities the child is focused on, the child may in turn comment back. The practitioner should recognize the caregiver's style and capitalize on it when teaching PoWRRS-Connect.

Family preferences can encompass quite a few aspects of the context related to PoWRRS-Connect. Preferences will be tied to style. Consider, for example, family members' preferences for how they spend their time and choose activities for their children. Some families may prefer being outside. Some might wish to play quietly indoors, reading books or doing art activities. Some families might love block building and pretend play, whereas others prefer unstructured social play with their children. Along with activities, preferences for types of toys or food need to be considered. Some families might like musical toys and love making lots of noise; other families might prefer pretend play with dolls. Knowing these preferences can be helpful when designing opportunities for PoWRRS-Connect. Another family preference might be time of day for implementing PoWRRS-Connect. Some families might find mealtime just too hectic for even thinking about using support strategies with their child, let alone applying the protocol, whereas others believe it ideal.

Considering the six elements of PoWRRS-Connect, practitioners should consider how the families view the protocol as a whole or in parts. Some families might find PoWRRS-Connect difficult to manage, or maybe they find particular elements quite easy and others hard, showing preference for one over others. For example, the first element of PoWRRS-Connect is provide an opportunity for communication. Caregivers have commented that offering children a choice of toys or snack items can easily be done throughout the day. Likewise, setting up opportunities for children to request more of an activity also seems to feel quite natural. This element has typically been easy to teach and is readily used by families. The elements of recognizing and responding are typically expected and thus might also be easier for caregivers to learn and use. However, many caregivers have commented that recognizing subtle child communication behaviors is sometimes difficult. Although responding is easy, describing what their child is doing requires some thought. Caregivers may need some extra instruction for these elements.

Our research has shown that shaping is the most difficult element to implement. This element urges the adult to elicit a more sophisticated, conventional form of behavior from the child when appropriate, which likely will be unusual for a caregiver. Deciding when to shape is the first decision; this requires reading the child and knowing if the timing is right for trying to elicit a different behavior. Furthermore, as practitioners know, successful shaping requires selecting the appropriate new behavior to elicit; one that is within reach for the child to produce. Finally, shaping requires deciding which prompts to use and administering them in an encouraging fashion to guide the child's effort. All of this makes shaping a difficult element to implement and one that families may avoid. Thus, practitioners should be aware that one or more elements of PoWRRS-Connect might need more instruction and encouragement than others.

Once preferences have been identified, practitioners will need to incorporate this information into their planning and actual instruction. As this chapter unfolds, as well as Chapter 8, practitioners will find specific ideas to facilitate the instruction of PoWRRS-Connect with caregivers, including elements that may be perceived as more difficult.

Child Characteristics

Using PoWRRS-Connect also requires understanding and appreciating a child's unique characteristics, including optimal states for engagement, positioning needs, learning style and preferences, and communication strengths and challenges. How these characteristics might influence using PoWRRS-Connect with families is described in the sections that follow.

States for Engagement   The best context for engaging and communicating with children, especially those with disabilities, demands that the child be truly ready to participate. *Readiness* includes several variables, including the child's state, positioning, learning style, and preferences for input. See Figure 7.2 for a description of infant states of consciousness from the Nursing Child Assessment Satellite Training (NCAST) at the University of Washington (NCAST, n.d.). State refers to a child's level of consciousness, typically described by two "sleep" states and four "wake" states. Sleep states include quiet sleep and active sleep. Wake states include a transition state of waking up or feeling drowsy, followed by quiet alert, active alert, and finally crying. In an ideal situation, the child should be in a quiet alert state, showing the child is receptive to adult input and eager to participate, whether it be feeding, talking, or playing. This would be the perfect time for PoWRRS-Connect.

Most families would recognize that sleep states, or making the transition from a sleep/drowsy state to being awake, are not a good time for learning. The active alert state typically occurs right before eating or when the child is ready for a change, such as repositioning,

The Six States of Consciousness

SLEEP STATES		
States	**Behaviors**	**Implications for Caregiving**
Quiet Sleep (non-REM)	Lack of body activity Smooth, regular respirations Lack of facial or eye movements Bursts of sucking movements Occasional startles Generally unresponsive	Very difficult to awaken. If awakened, quickly returns to sleep. Good time for activities that require little or no body movement or response, e.g., trimming fingernails. Intrusive procedures not recommended. Feeding will be unsuccessful.
Active Sleep (REM)	More body activity Irregular respirations Movements of face, may smile Movement of eyes under the lids More responsive to stimuli	Easier to awaken. Parents may think baby is awake. Feeding will be unsuccessful.
TRANSITIONAL STATE		
Drowsy	Variable activity Irregular respirations Opens and closes eyes Eyes glazed, heavy-lidded look Delayed responsiveness	More easy to awaken. Difficult to tell if babies are awake or asleep. If left alone, babies may go back to sleep. Take time to fully awaken before feeding. To awaken, give babies something to see, hear, or suck.
AWAKE STATES		
Quiet Alert	Minimal body activity Regular respirations Face has bright, shiny look Eyes wide and bright Most attentive to stimuli	Good time to feed, talk, look at, or hold the infant. Baby will respond and learn best in this state. In the first few hours after birth, most newborns have intense periods of this state, followed by a long sleep period.
Active Alert	Much body activity Irregular respirations Facial movement Eyes open but not bright Fussiness Sensitive to stimuli	State in which most babies begin feeding. Beginning signal for a change, e.g., need to be fed, repositioned, and so on. May be difficult to get the infant to interact. If left alone in this state, baby will often begin attempts to self-console.
Crying	Irregular respirations Facial grimace Cries Color changes Variable sensitivity to stimuli	Baby's limits have been reached. Signals a need for a change. May attempt to console self. Will most likely need consoling by caregiver.

Figure 7.2.   The six states of consciousness. (From Nursing Child Assessment Satellite Training [NCAST], University of Washington School of Nursing. [n.d.]. The Six States of Consciousness [course handout]. Reprinted by permission.)

or a new activity. It might be difficult to get the child's full attention at this moment. This might be a time when the adult needs to step in to assist the child in changing focus; practitioners should be prepared to provide families with some ideas for doing this.

Note that for some children with severe disabilities, state may be hard to discern, or it may be quite variable. Some children may have their wake states compromised for medical reasons (e.g., seizures, medication), particularly varying from day to day. Other children may be easily agitated, quietly alert one moment and fussing or crying another. The practitioner will naturally need to work closely with families to decide optimum times for interjecting PoWRRS-Connect into everyday routines.

Positioning   All children need to have adequate positioning for participating in interactions with others. They need to see the adult and any items that are being presented. For children with severe motor impairments, positioning is exceptionally important to consider when implementing PoWRRS-Connect. Motor therapists (physical therapist or occupational therapist) will play a critical role in providing input about adjusting and maintaining positioning for optimum communication. Engagement and communication take place throughout the day, and sometimes positioning will not be ideal. As with the child's state, consider positioning for implementing PoWRRS-Connect and the particular activity that is occurring. Some positioning guidelines for interacting during mealtime, or playing with toys or social games, follow:

- The goal is positioning that maximizes postural stability and alignment as the foundation for interactive play with the child.

- Positioning may be best achieved by adapting current seating using foam inserts or other supportive equipment.

- Positioning also may be best achieved through new seating that better fits the child and enables the child to more actively participate in the play and social interaction.

- The position of the adult is of equal importance. The adult should be positioned at the child's eye level and at midline to maximize engagement and communication.

Good positioning and seating can be described by the following checkpoints:

- Pelvis at 90 degrees

- Trunk upright and stable

- Feet firmly supported

- Head (and eyes) in midline

- Shoulders or arms forward

- Arms free to reach

Figure 7.3 provides photos of a child in two sitting positions. This child has very low tone, exacerbated by poor positioning. Note in the first photo how the child literally seems to melt into the chair. The positioning is not supporting his motor needs. He is sitting back on his pelvis (posterior tilt), reducing his overall stability. Without pelvic stability and alignment, the child lacks the trunk support to sit up and instead flops to the side. This in turn reduces head and neck support and prevents him from being able to lift his head. Note, too, that the tray is too high, which prevents him from seeing toys; plus, the lip

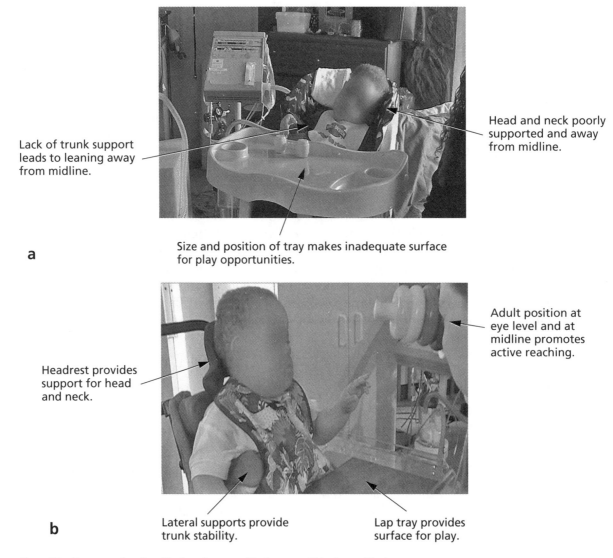

Lack of trunk support leads to leaning away from midline.

Head and neck poorly supported and away from midline.

Size and position of tray makes inadequate surface for play opportunities.

a

Adult position at eye level and at midline promotes active reaching.

Headrest provides support for head and neck.

b

Lateral supports provide trunk stability.

Lap tray provides surface for play.

Figure 7.3. Two examples of positioning: a) poor positioning versus b) better positioning.

on the tray requires him to lift his arm—an impossible task! The second photo illustrates the same child one week later in a new chair. Look at the difference! He still has low tone but with better positioning his motor abilities are maximized. His pelvis is positioned and supported at 90 degrees so that his trunk is both aligned and more upright. His head is supported upright and with his pelvis and trunk supported, he can maintain his body and head in midline. The tray is at a lower height, and there is no lip, so he can reach forward and play. Supporting the improved positioning is the adult, who is seated midline and at his eye level, which in turn helps the child maintain good head positioning and facilitates interaction. The difference in positioning for this child was monumental and revealed that he had more engagement and communication skills than originally thought.

Sometimes positioning for engagement and communication is optimal when two adults are involved with the child during an interaction. One adult serves to assist with positioning, whereas the other adult maintains the interaction. For children with severe motor impairments, this setup often occurs in co-treatment sessions. Co-treatment refers to a motor therapist (e.g., PT, OT) working with another therapist or family member to optimize a child's positioning for learning during treatment. It can serve as an excellent way to maximize a child's performance. Appendix C provides an overview of an excellent video that illustrates the implementation and benefits of co-treatment (see **Video 3, Benjamin**).

Style and Preferences Child styles and preferences will also need to be considered when implementing PoWRRS-Connect. Style refers to the child's temperament and learning approach. Temperament is often depicted by several different personal traits and reflects a child's activity level, adaptability to surroundings, sensitivity and intensity of reactions, and distractibility versus persistence. Children can be described as easy or flexible, active or feisty, or slow to warm or cautious. Other children might be seen as impulsive versus reflective. A child's temperament is not written in stone, and on any given day or at any given time, the child's temperament can vary, becoming more or less obvious. In addition, for some children with disabilities, determining style might be challenging, similar to determining state. However, as the practitioner considers a family's implementation of PoWRRS-Connect, knowing a child's general tendencies in style can help appreciate the ease or difficulty with which the protocol might be used. For example, for a child who appears impulsive, the practitioner might give the caregiver ideas for helping their child attend when presenting communication opportunities. For a child who appears more reflective, the practitioner might point out the importance of waiting and giving the child ample time to respond. Another aspect of temperament is how well the child can regulate their behavior. Some children find it easy to transition from one activity to the next, whereas other children find transitions difficult. Families will likely be sensitive to this quality, and practitioners can provide tips for implementing the PoWRRS-Connect protocol to children's styles.

Another important consideration is how well the caregiver's style matches the child's style. For example, a caregiver who is talkative and enjoys lots of stimulation, such as textured materials, bright lights, or lots of music, may find it more difficult identifying the best toys for their child who is easily distracted and gets fussy when overstimulated. Another aspect of style addresses how children best learn. Some children are quiet, passive learners who tend to prefer watching and gathering information at their own pace. Other children are more active learners; they are risk takers and often are imitators. For the former group, no amount of prompting or cuing will get the child to imitate; these children will do it when they are ready. For this group, a lot of modeling and hand-over-hand guidance can be valuable in stimulating communication and new behaviors. Showing these children options and encouraging their efforts goes a long way. The more active/risk-takers group seem to want to try anything new and different. They will often spontaneously imitate gestures and even vocalizations. No one style is better than another; the fun lies in recognizing and appreciating style differences.

As can be seen, style leads to preferences. Children's style often will dictate their preferences in activities, toy selection, and food choices. A child who shows sensitivity to stimulation might find a loud or surprising toy frightening. This same child might love smooth surfaces and hate textured ones. Some children prefer motion toys, whereas others prefer toys that light up. Paying attention to a child's preferences can make or break an activity. In PoWRRS-Connect, this child characteristic is particularly important to consider when providing opportunities for communication. When setting up a choice opportunity, knowing a child's preference can be valuable in offering a preferred versus a nonpreferred item. When setting up a request opportunity, particularly requesting "more," using a preferred item almost guarantees success. Discovering a child's preferences will likely require trial

Table 7.2. Child style and preferences

Style

- Flexible versus rigid
- Active versus passive
- Attentive versus distractible
- Sensory seeking versus sensory avoiding

Preferences

- Types of activities and activity locations
- Types of toys
- Types of food
- Times of day

and error. Sometimes it takes implementing PoWRRS-Connect to reveal this information. Table 7.2 presents a brief list of child styles and preferences to consider before implementing PoWRRS-Connect.

Communication Skills: Which Behaviors to Emphasize   Children will present with communication skills and abilities that fall at different places along the continuum of communication behaviors that was introduced in Chapter 1 and re-presented in Figure 7.4. Research has shown that optimum learning takes place when instruction recognizes where the child is currently functioning (**actual level of performance**) and where they can perform with assistance from others (**potential level of performance**) (Feuerstein et al., 1979).

Preintentional

Single focus: looking and sustaining gaze to a person OR an object
- Gaze alone
- Gaze + gestures OR vocalizations
- Gaze + gestures AND vocalizations

Dual focus: looking from an object to a person OR a person to an object
- Gaze alone
- Gaze + gestures OR vocalizations
- Gaze + gestures AND vocalizations

Triadic focus: looking back and forth between an object and a person (person-object-person OR object-person-object)
- Gaze alone
- Gaze + gestures OR vocalizations
- Gaze + gestures AND vocalizations

Intentional

Figure 7.4. Preverbal communication behaviors: Foundation for first words. (Adapted from Brady et al., 2012. Republished with permission of American Speech-Language-Hearing Association, from Development of the Communication Complexity Scale, Brady, N., Fleming, K., Thiemann-Bourke, K, Olswang, L., Dowden, P., & Saunders, M., *21*, 1, 2012; permission conveyed through Copyright Clearance Center, Inc.)

When using PoWRRS-Connect, the practitioner will want to understand both the child's actual and potential levels of performance, with regards to their use of preverbal communication behaviors along the communication continuum. The behaviors that the child routinely produces without guidance (actual) describe where to start with PoWRRS-Connect. The behaviors that the child is able to produce with prompts and support from an adult (potential) show the practitioner how to plan for using PoWRRS-Connect and what change to expect. For children who are easily stimulated to produce new behaviors with prompts, change is highly anticipated. For children who show more difficulty in producing behaviors with prompts and cues, change is likely going to be slower. To facilitate the best outcomes, practitioners should know which behaviors show the best potential for learning and which prompts best facilitate desired outcomes. Consider, for example, the child profiles of Sophie, Jack, and Amelia presented in Chapter 5. Some children immediately will be ready to work on producing a full, three-point triadic gaze with or without accompanying gestures and vocalizations. Others may require support on some of the communication and engagement behaviors that serve as a foundation for later production of triadic gaze.

When partnering with families, practitioners will need to have a good sense of the child's actual and potential communication behaviors and the prompts that seem most promising. The Checklist of Early Communication Behaviors (hereafter referred to as Checklist), introduced in Chapter 5, will serve as the guide for making this determination and for explaining to families how to best use the PoWRRS-Connect protocol. Part 2 of this chapter discusses how to use the Checklist to identify the child's actual and potential levels of performance in conversation with the family.

Keeping in mind the family and child characteristics described previously, the remainder of this chapter walks the practitioner through using PoWRRS-Connect with families during the first visit, which typically follows evaluation and assessment. This first visit often lays the foundation for the practitioner–caregiver partnership, as each works together to accomplish the family's IFSP goals and objectives. Because a coaching paradigm currently is a predominant approach in service delivery for infants and toddlers, suggestions for instructing families are offered using coaching techniques (e.g., observe, model, practice, reflect, plan) familiar to many practitioners.

PART 2: IMPLEMENTING PoWRRS-CONNECT WITH FAMILIES—THE FIRST VISIT

The second part of this chapter takes the practitioner step by step through a typical first visit in which PoWRRS-Connect is implemented with a child and their family. The overall structure of the first visit may feel quite familiar to practitioners—this is intentional. Using the PoWRRS-Connect protocol with families should integrate rather seamlessly with strategies commonly used in early support services and the instructional practices recommended by the Division for Early Childhood (DEC; 2014).

At the beginning of the first visit, the practitioner and family should briefly review the family's IFSP goals to get the team focusing on the same priorities. Next, the practitioner and caregivers together will identify an authentic routine or activity that is fun and motivating for the caregiver and the child. This routine or activity provides the context for service delivery. Before jumping into using PoWRRS-Connect, the practitioner and caregivers will discuss the child's current level of functioning and agree on appropriate early communication behaviors to target. Finally, the practitioner will introduce the

PoWRRS-Connect protocol with families to move from the child's actual to potential level of functioning.

Figure 7.5 provides a schematic of the general steps the practitioner and family will move through during the first visit in which PoWRRS-Connect is used as well as a list of supporting materials for each step. The sections that follow take the reader through each step and provide examples of how the steps may unfold using the profile of Sophie, first introduced in Chapter 5.

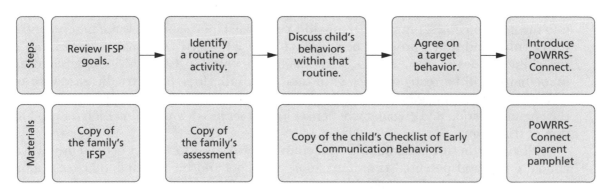

Figure 7.5.   Outline of the first visit using PoWRRS-Connect, with supporting materials. (*Key*, IFSP, individualized family service plan.)

Review the IFSP Goals

The first visit with a family that follows the evaluation and assessment process should begin with reviewing the family's IFSP goals. The IFSP goals highlight the family's priorities for their child and should serve as a guide for each visit. Many IFSP goals will center around supporting the child's independence, communication, and social engagement within and across the family's authentic everyday routines and activities. TGI and the six essential elements of the PoWRRS-Connect protocol offer one powerful approach that can be used to support children and families in accomplishing their goals. Practitioners should begin the first visit by reading the IFSP goals aloud with the family. The family may identify which goal is a priority for that visit.

Consider the following example from Chapter 5: Sophie's family reported a desire to help her play with her siblings (social engagement) by taking a turn (communication, independence) rather than passively watching the older children play together. One of Sophie's IFSP goals focuses on supporting Sophie to request a turn by teaching her specific conventional communication behaviors: looking at a toy and reaching. Reviewing this IFSP goal with the family at the start of the visit helps to position the behavioral objective (looking + reaching) within a meaningful goal identified by the family (taking a turn) as a priority. Spending just a few minutes reviewing the IFSP goals with the family at the onset of the first visit, and at subsequent visits, provides the opportunity for the practitioner to remind the family that PoWRRS-Connect will help them accomplish these goals.

Identify an Authentic Routine or Activity

Once the IFSP goals have been reviewed with the family and one goal has been selected as a priority for the visit, the next step is to identify an authentic routine or activity that can be used to address this goal. Recall that the practitioner should introduce PoWRRS-Connect within a routine that the family identifies as relatively fun and easy, versus stressful and hard. Integrating PoWRRS-Connect into service delivery will be new for the practitioner, the family, and the child. Beginning with a routine that is fun, easy, and motivating to the child and family will set the practitioner and caregivers up for success.

Continuing with Sophie's example, the family previously identified a daily routine that offers an opportunity to work on supporting Sophie's early communication and independence. Recall that each day, before her siblings get on the school bus, the children spend about 10 minutes playing together. This routine is one that occurs consistently during the week, is of appropriate duration for Sophie's attention, is a fun and relaxing time for the family, and offers the opportunity for Sophie and her caregivers to focus on one specific behavioral objective: using gaze and gestures (reaching) to work toward the goal of Sophie using gaze and gestures to request a turn during a meaningful activity (playing with her siblings).

Discuss the Child's Current Behaviors (Actual)

Before beginning to work on a specific communication behavior (or behaviors), it is important that the family and the practitioner agree about how the child is currently functioning within the chosen routine or activity. Returning to the Checklist, first introduced during the assessment, will help guide the conversation about the child's current, or actual, level of communication functioning. The practitioner should present the Checklist and review the types of conventional communication behaviors (gaze, gestures, and/or vocalizations) that were either reported by the family or directly observed by the practitioner during the initial assessment. Both the practitioner and the family will benefit from being reminded of their ideas about the child's actual skills and abilities. Depending on the duration of time between completion of the Checklist and the first visit, the child may have gained (or lost) skills. Acknowledging and recording such changes will be important. Reviewing this Checklist also provides an excellent opportunity to reorient the practitioner–caregiver team to the child's current strengths and challenges.

Reminder: Bring a copy of the IFSP Goal and the Checklist of Early Communication Behaviors to the first visit!

The Checklist also may be used to help the practitioner and family discuss the child's behaviors across contexts. Often, children present with inconsistencies in skills across settings, activities, communication partners, and times of day (as discussed previously in this chapter with regard to different states of engagement). Families may provide rich information about the variability they observe in their children across such contexts. The practitioner can make notes on the communication Checklist that highlight the different contexts in which a child is best able to show their most sophisticated skills and those in which communication and social engagement can be more challenging.

Finally, when reviewing the Checklist, the practitioner and caregiver may have different ideas about the child's skills. This first visit offers an opportunity to openly discuss any discrepancies between the two perspectives. These conversations are critical to building a strong foundation for the practitioner–caregiver partnership. Caregivers may offer insight about the child's skills that the practitioner may not have yet had the opportunity to observe and vice versa. The practitioner and family do not have to agree on the child's current level of functioning, but as many practitioners already know, understanding and acknowledging each other's perspectives is an important part of building a productive working relationship. The minutes spent reviewing the Checklist during the first visit will be well spent as they offer the chance to recalibrate with the family and reorient the family to the developmental sequence of early communication behaviors that will be addressed through TGI. Once the child's current level of functioning is determined, the practitioner and family may begin to plan the session based on an appropriate next step along the communication continuum.

For Sophie, the practitioner and the family agreed that paying attention to people (vs. objects) is one of Sophie's strengths. Using the Checklist, the assessment documented that she is independently sustaining a single focus as described along the communication continuum. Thus, Sophie's actual level of performance can be described as sustaining gaze to people.

Select a Target Behavior (Potential)

The practitioner also needs to know which preverbal communication behaviors (gaze, gestures, vocalizations) are in reach for the child when support is provided (potential level of performance). These are the behaviors that can be produced when adults provide prompts (i.e., verbal, visual, auditory, tactile support). This describes where the child is headed through PoWRRS-Connect. Based on the previous conversations, the practitioner and family together pick a target behavior (or behaviors) from the communication continuum (shown on the Checklist) that is just one step beyond what the child is currently doing in the chosen context.

Consider Sophie and her family again. Sophie independently is sustaining gaze to people but often gets "stuck" on faces. With support, Sophie can shift her gaze from a communication partner to a shared object or toy during a play routine (dual focus). This ability to shift gaze from person to object (or object to person) is a building block toward triadic gaze production. Given that Sophie is stimulable for this behavior but is not yet producing it independently, gaze shifts from people to objects would be an appropriate target behavior to integrate into PoWRRS-Connect for Sophie. Selecting a target behavior that is within reach will help the family work toward building the potential for Sophie's independence and communicative competence during fun and motivating play routines with her siblings.

Use the PoWRRS-Connect Protocol to Move From Actual to Potential

The following sections describe the steps for using PoWRRS-Connect with families during daily routines and activities to help children move from their actual level of performance in production of preverbal communication behaviors to their potential level of performance. These steps—observe, model, practice, reflect, and plan—likely will be familiar to many practitioners working with infants and toddlers who use a coaching approach with families. The steps are borrowed from a coaching model (Rush & Sheldon, 2011, 2020) but adapted and discussed next as they will guide practitioners instructing families to use PoWRRS-Connect.

Observe   Implementing PoWRRS-Connect begins by observing the family interacting with their child in the routine or activity that was identified at the beginning of the session, as described previously. By simply observing the caregiver and child interact, the practitioner has an opportunity to note what is working well, what is challenging, and how the child is functioning. The practitioner may begin by saying, "I want to watch how this routine typically goes for you. Show me how you and your child typically [insert activity here]." As the caregiver and child interact, the practitioner should make note of how the caregiver sets up the routine or activity, which behaviors the child produces (gaze, gesture, vocalization), and how the caregiver responds. The goal of this observation is to identify what is working well and to provide positive feedback to the caregiver. For example, the practitioner may point out to the family which parts of the PoWRRS-Connect cycle are already naturally present in the caregiver–child interaction. If none of the PoWRRS-Connect elements is part of the caregiver–child interaction, that is okay, too. The practitioner simply makes a note of this and finds something positive to comment on. It can be as simple as observing that the caregiver is using a positive tone and/or positive affect with their child or as specific as noting a part of the PoWRRS-Connect cycle that is already in use by the caregiver. It also is important to comment on the behaviors that the child uses when interacting with their caregivers. The practitioner can note which behaviors she observes the child producing and refer back to the communication Checklist that was previously reviewed.

Model   After observing the caregiver and child interaction, the practitioner picks one or two elements within the PoWRRS-Connect cycle to model while the caregiver watches. Some caregivers may wish to jot down notes about what the practitioner does and how their child responds. Others may ask to video the practitioner so they can review the strategies later. As discussed earlier in this chapter, each family's learning styles and preferences will be different. The practitioner should be ready and willing to adapt to the different preferences and needs of individual families.

At first, the practitioner should keep the model as simple as possible to ensure that the caregiver experiences success when it is their turn to try. Some caregivers will need to focus on one element of the PoWRRS-Connect cycle at a time. Others may be ready to link elements together as the interaction unfolds between the caregiver and the child. It is up to the practitioner to use their clinical expertise and experience when deciding how much to model for the caregiver. Regardless of the amount of modeling provided, the practitioner should be clear and explicit about what she is doing. Narrating each step as it unfolds will be important to make each step explicit, as caregivers learn new ways of interacting with their child.

Practice   After a model is provided, the caregiver then takes a turn trying the element(s) of PoWRRS-Connect demonstrated by the practitioner. As the caregiver interacts with their child, the practitioner will give feedback in the moment to support the caregiver in achieving success. In early sessions, or when a component is brand new to a caregiver, the practitioner may be providing a lot of in-the-moment support. In later sessions, as the caregiver feels more confident and competent, the practitioner may offer less in-the-moment support. Again, the caregiver's learning preferences and styles should be considered when supporting families to implement PoWRRS-Connect elements in natural routines or activities. Some families may benefit from being provided with explicit and frequent instructions as they interact with their child; others may wish to try on their own with little upfront input. As the practitioner and the caregiver work together to support the child, it is important to be open and transparent about what works (and what does not) for each family. Understanding and honoring the family's preferences will help build a true partnership between the practitioner and the family.

To illustrate modeling and practice, **Video 7.1, Working With Parent: Modeling and Practice,** illustrates a practitioner (Dr. Gay Lloyd Pinder) working with the father of a little boy, who is learning to use gaze to engage, specifically to look at his father, not just the toy.

Note the position of Dad and practitioner, both close and at eye level with the child. Dad is positioned more at midline than the practitioner, who is off to the side offering suggestions. Also note the consistent positive feedback the practitioner is providing Dad as he plays with his son. This video also illustrates the value of play. The rings are an excellent toy of choice for this child, easy to hold and, more important, the ring itself provides a visual focus for the child to look at and through to his dad's eye. This toy, and the interaction around it, allows the emphasis to be on helping the child shift his gaze from the ring to his dad, particularly focusing on eyes. Note particularly the lovely shift between the use of the ring to draw eye contact and then back to play as the child explores putting his hand through the ring. Throughout the video, the practitioner is both modeling and supporting Dad's efforts to play with and teach his son, who is fully engaged throughout. The child is learning about objects, gaze, engagement, and communication, all within a play context. This video segment not only illustrates modeling and practice, but it also provides a wonderful illustration of administering the shaping element in PoWRRS-Connect.

Reflect   After the caregiver practices implementing one or more of the PoWRRS-Connect elements with the child, the practitioner and caregiver should pause and debrief about how that practice felt. The practitioner can begin by asking a simple, open-ended question, "What about that felt like it went well or was natural for you? What was more challenging or felt less natural?" The caregiver's responses to these questions set the stage for a reflection about how PoWRRS-Connect is working. As the caregiver thinks and reflects, the practitioner provides feedback—both supportive and constructive. The conversation should always begin with supportive feedback that identifies at least one thing the caregiver has done well, which helps build confidence and competence. Constructive feedback is meant to offer ideas and opportunities for adjustments that will only further support the child's and caregiver's success. During this conversation, the practitioner and caregiver will also brainstorm about what works for the specific child.

Plan   Finally, each session should end with a plan for what the caregiver and child will do between visits. The plan should be a concrete set of steps or actions that the caregiver will try before the practitioner and family meet again. Note that making a plan is not the same as assigning homework for the family. The plan should be a joint effort between the practitioner and caregiver that can easily be tackled during the family's everyday routines and activities. For example, the practitioner and family should identify one routine that will happen with some regularity in the upcoming days and identify one, more, or all of the specific PoWRRS-Connect elements that the caregiver will implement during this routine.

To help the family use PoWRRS-Connect between visits with the practitioner, a family handout is provided in Appendix D; it is also available on the Brookes Download Hub with the other downloadable resources for this book. This handout presents each of the six essential elements of the PoWRRS-Connect protocol discussed in Chapter 6 (provide opportunity, wait, recognize, respond, shape, connect) but in an easy-to-digest format with accompanying visuals for families. It also includes a table illustrating ideas for how to implement PoWRRS-Connect during play with their children. This handout, available in English and Spanish, should be presented as a resource for families and may be introduced in conjunction with the "stick to the six!" mantra described in Chapter 6. Families may wish to leave a copy of the handout in places within their home where they typically engage in the routines and activities in which they will be using PoWRRS-Connect.

CONCLUSION

This chapter, presented in two parts, discussed how to put the PoWRRS-Connect protocol into action with families and children. Part 1 introduced both family and child characteristics that should be considered before implementing PoWRRS-Connect in a visit. Variations in families' and children's styles, preferences, skills, and abilities should all be considered as practitioners partner with caregivers in using PoWRRS-Connect to support children in reaching their potential. Part 2 provided step-by-step guidance for introducing PoWRRS-Connect during the first visit with a family after evaluation and assessment. After reading Chapters 6 and 7, practitioners should have a clear idea of how to introduce and implement the six essential elements of the PoWRRS-Connect protocol. Chapter 8 will provide tips for tailoring TGI and PoWRRS-Connect to meet individual child and family needs and offer suggestions for troubleshooting when challenges arise.

CHAPTER 8

Tips for Tailoring Triadic Gaze Intervention and PoWRRS-Connect With Families

Implementing TGI in service delivery can be exciting but also a bit overwhelming. Chapter 5 described how to decide if TGI is a good fit for a family's needs and priorities. Chapter 6 provided details regarding the administration of PoWRRS-Connect. Chapter 7 walked the practitioner through a first visit with a family using the PoWRRS-Connect protocol. This chapter provides practitioners with tips for tailoring TGI to meet the individual and often varied needs of children and families during the administration of PoWRRS-Connect. The chapter should help answer questions that may arise once practitioners are using PoWRRS-Connect regularly. Although the steps for implementing the PoWRRS-Connect protocol have been presented as a relatively straightforward process, practitioners know that implementing any protocol rarely proceeds according to plan. Practitioners inevitably will need to adjust their delivery of the PoWRRS-Connect protocol to meet the individual differences across children, accommodate cultural variations among families, and adapt to changes that children and families make over time. The content that composes this chapter shares some of the collective experience and wisdom gathered over years of TGI implementation in both research and clinical contexts. The videos described in Chapters 6 and 7 and Appendix C should be helpful in appreciating how PoWRRS-Connect can be tailored to individual children and families.

This chapter begins where Chapter 7 left off: discussing how the PoWRRS-Connect protocol becomes integrated into a family's everyday routines and activities. Although this topic was introduced in Chapters 4 and 6, this chapter offers specific ideas to help practitioners support families in feeling confident and competent at making the PoWRRS-Connect elements a natural part of everyday interactions with their children. This includes consideration for recognizing and honoring a family's cultural context. Next, the chapter provides tips for establishing and maintaining child engagement during communication opportunities, describing adjustments that might be required when working with children with CCN. Special attention is paid to the properties of toys (or everyday objects that can be used as toys) and how toys can be used to maximize engagement. The chapter then turns to offering advice for considering individual children's skills and abilities, including suggestions for what to do when a child's skills do not quite fit along the continuum of communication behavior described in this book. Finally, the chapter concludes with ideas for helping the practitioner talk with families about how to fine-tune shaping their children's signals.

MAKING PoWRRS-CONNECT A NATURAL PART OF CAREGIVER–CHILD INTERACTIONS

When integrating TGI into a family's IFSP, the hope is that over time and with support from the practitioner, families will begin to view the PoWRRS-Connect elements as a natural way to interact with their children. For this to happen, PoWRRS-Connect must fit into the everyday activities, routines, and simple moments that arise across a family's day. Specific ideas for how to accomplish this are included in the first section that follows. The family also must see the value in adopting PoWRRS-Connect as a new approach and build confidence in using the PoWRRS-Connect elements when interacting with their children. The important role that the practitioner plays in supporting caregiver confidence and competence is discussed in the second section that follows. Finally, families present with different strengths, needs, priorities, cultural practices, and resources. As practitioners acknowledge and respect such variations across families, they will need to come up with ways to embrace families' needs as they encourage the use of PoWRRS-Connect. The third section that follows provides some guidance in that regard.

Embedding Communication Opportunities Into Authentic Routines Throughout the Day

Chapter 7 presented ideas for talking with families about their daily routines and activities. Identifying specific moments for integrating PoWRRS-Connect into a family's life requires a deep understanding of their day-to-day, authentic routines. Some families will freely and easily outline their daily schedule with the practitioner, providing enough detail for the practitioner to identify moments in which communication opportunities may be presented to the child. Other families initially may be less forthcoming or may require more support to see the multitude of moments that arise across a typical day, which present opportunities for using the PoWRRS-Connect protocol. Table 8.1 provides some examples of common family routines and ideas for embedding communication opportunities (both choice and request) into the family's day. These routines begin with waking up and starting the day and end with putting the child to bed at night. Specific ideas are presented for routines referenced in previous chapters (e.g., mealtimes, bath time, bedtime).

Some Tips for Implementing PoWRRS-Connect

PoWRRS-Connect should be a natural part of interactions with children.
- Embed communication opportunities in authentic routines.
- Support caregivers' confidence and competence.
- Respect and embrace family differences.

Children's engagement is key.
- Ensure communication opportunities stand out.
- Be aware of children's vision and possible challenges.
- Make the most of all kinds of toys (and objects that can be toys).

Children do not always move smoothly through the developing communication continuum.
Shaping will need to be tailored to individual children.
- Select prompts to match child style and preferences.
- Consider when to shape and when not to shape.
- Weigh the number of prompts to give.

Table 8.1. Tips for embedding communication opportunities into typical family routines and activities throughout the day

	Opportunity type	
	Choice	Request
Typical family routine	*Offer choices between. . . .*	*Pause during the routine and allow the child to ask for "more. . ."*
Waking up or starting the day	• Steps for opening the family home for the day (e.g., turning on the lights or opening the curtains first)	• Verses of a favorite good morning song
Eating a meal or snack	• Food items • Drinks • Plates, cups, or utensils placed at the table or on the highchair	• Bites of a favorite food • Sips of a favorite drink
Getting ready for the day	• Activities to do first (e.g., brush hair, brush teeth) • Items of clothing (e.g., two options for shirts, pants, socks, etc.) • Which item of clothing to put on first	• Brushing (hair or teeth) • Socks or shoes (i.e., second sock or shoe to be put on the other foot)
Leaving the apartment or house	• Toys or books to take on the car ride or walk • Which item to put in the diaper bag	• Heading out the door—pause by the closed door in the middle of leaving and wait for the child to indicate "more" (e.g., "Open the door!")
Leaving child (at child care; with grandparents, family members, or neighbor) when caregiver goes to work	• Ways to greet teachers, friends, a grandparent, a family member, or a neighbor (wave, high-five, silly dance) • Which toy or activity center to explore first	• Hello to teachers, friends, a grandparent, a family member, or a neighbor—after helping the child say hello to one caregiver or friend, pause for a request to say hello to the next caregiver or friend.
Picking up child (from child care, grandparents, family members, or neighbor) when caregiver returns from work	• Ways to say goodbye to teachers, friends, a grandparent, a family member, or a neighbor (examples above) • Which toys to put away first	• (See example above for "Leaving the apartment or house")
Doing the laundry	• Which item of laundry goes into the washer or dryer next—make a fun game of throwing the item into the machine	• Tosses of items into the machine • Soap to the washing machine—make a fun game of pouring it in slowly then pausing for the child
Feeding or taking care of the family pet	• Which bowl to fill first (e.g., food, water) • Which toy to play with (e.g., ball, chew toy)	• Scoops of food into the pet's food dish • Brushes for the pet
Walking the dog	• Which toy to take along on the walk • Which direction to go on the walk	• Moving or walking—create a stop or go game; child asks for more "go"
Going for a walk	• Ways to walk (or be pushed) (e.g., slow vs. fast) • Which direction to go • Whose hand to hold (if walking) • Who pushes the stroller or wheelchair • Which snacks and/or toys to take along	• Pushes in the stroller—adult can play the "stop and go" game
Taking a bath	• Which toys to bring into the tub • Which washcloth to use (e.g., washcloth vs. sponge) • Which body parts to wash first (e.g., head vs. hands vs. feet)	• Tickles in the tub while washing up • Singing while washing (e.g., "This is the way we wash our feet, wash our feet, wash our feet. . .")
Reading books	• Which book to read	• Turning the page
Cleaning up the apartment or house	• Which activity to do first (e.g., wipe table or vacuum floors)	• Putting in or emptying items from the dishwasher • Wiping up the table • Squirts of window cleaner on the windows
Going to the park	• Which equipment to play on (e.g., swings vs. slide) • Who gives pushes on the swings (e.g., mom, dad, big sister or brother, abuela)	• Pushes on the swing • Turns down the slide
Going shopping at the grocery (or other) store	• Which item to put in the cart	• Pushes in the cart down the aisle
Going to bed	• Which jammies to wear • Which lovey, stuffed animal, or blankie to bring to bed	• Goodnight kisses, hugs, or snuggles

For example, caregivers can embed communication at mealtime by offering a choice between two food items or setting up an opportunity to request more of a favorite food or drink. Additional ideas for routines selected from our work with families over the years are also included. For example, some families enlist the help of their children to accomplish daily household chores. These often seemingly mundane tasks offer opportunities to use the PoWRRS-Connect protocol for communication and engagement. Consider, for example, doing the laundry; all items in the laundry basket must eventually make their way into the washing machine or dryer. The caregiver can make a game of putting items into the machine with the child by holding up two items of clothing, asking the child which item goes in "next," and then tossing that item (or allowing the child to toss the item) into the machine in a fun and spirited way. As an alternative, the caregiver may hold all the items of clothing and allow the child to toss the items in one by one. The caregiver can then pause and present a request opportunity by withholding the next item of clothing until the child indicates, through gaze, gesture, and/or vocalization, that the child wants another turn to toss an item into the machine.

Tips such as those offered in Table 8.1 are by no means exhaustive. They are meant to serve as a resource for practitioners and families as they begin to discuss when and how to embed opportunities for communication into the family's authentic routines. The PoWRRS-Connect protocol should integrate seamlessly into a family's day and not present extra work for the family. Caregivers already face an immense and important job in caring for their children; PoWRRS-Connect should enhance the caregiver–child interactions that are naturally occurring. Practitioners will need to assess a family's typical routines and consider how PoWRRS-Connect can easily fit into what caregivers naturally are doing. Table 8.1 and also the PoWRRS-Connect caregiver handout in Appendix D provide some ideas for practitioners, but of course, individual families' day-to-day interactions must be considered and valued as practitioners encourage caregivers to use PoWRRS-Connect.

Supporting Caregiver Confidence and Competence

As conversations about embedding PoWRRS-Connect into everyday routines unfold, the practitioner must acknowledge that asking families to integrate the protocol into these everyday moments may require that they learn new ways of interacting with their children. Changing a family's interaction patterns, even in small and incremental ways, can be challenging. Engaging children with CCN may come easily to some families, whereas others may have a history of difficult experiences or failed attempts at communicating with their children. In either scenario, it is likely that many families fall into habitual patterns of interacting with their children—some useful and others less so. Introducing new ideas through the PoWRRS-Connect protocol may be a welcome change for some but may be met by resistance by others.

Regardless of the family's perspective, all caregivers need to believe that they are capable of supporting their children's communication. The PoWRRS-Connect protocol is meant to enhance the positive things that families are already doing as they interact with their children. To best support families, the practitioner should always begin from a position of presumed competence. The practitioner should highlight what families are already doing to support their child during simple moments of engagement. No accomplishment is too small. The practitioner might comment, for example, "Wow, when you look at José and smile, his whole body gets quiet, like he's really listening to what you're saying even if he's not looking at you with his eyes!" As the practitioner brings these subtle, positive moments of engagement, however fleeting, to the forefront, the family begins from a position of strength. When families feel that they are competent and capable, they likely will be more motivated to try something new with their children.

Families also need to believe that the effort they put forth in using the PoWRRS-Connect protocol is worth the payoff. To reinforce this point, the practitioner should emphasize the connect part of PoWRRS-Connect. The elements that compose the protocol ultimately serve to build moments of connection between parent and child. Social engagement and communication flow from these everyday moments of connection. When using the PoWRRS-Connect protocol with families, the practitioner should stress the power of connection as the foundation for every interaction. The remainder of the elements are used to expand those moments of sustained engagement and build the child's communication skills. Connection likely already exists between parent and child in some form. The practitioner's job is to bring this connection to the forefront at each visit and use it as a foundation on which to embed PoWRRS-Connect.

Acknowledging and Respecting Variations Across Families

Thus far, the caregiver–child connection has been emphasized. However, it is important to acknowledge that family constellations are varied and dynamic. Practitioners need to recognize, respect, and honor the differences between and among families as they share ideas for supporting the child and family. Differences can be as varied as the families, including who assumes the role of primary caregiver, who makes decisions within the family unit, how the adult–child interaction styles unfold, and which activities and routines are used. For example, in some family units, the practitioner may be working primarily with a mother–child dyad. In other family units, the central dyad may consist of a child and the grandmother, aunt, father, grandfather, or any one of a myriad of other possible adult–child combinations, and even older child–younger child caregiving arrangements. These different constellations will likely consist of multiple styles and conventions. Each adult–child dyad is unique and will require consideration by the practitioner as they begin to interact with and support families in using PoWRRS-Connect.

Just as family constellations and dynamics vary, so too will preferences for activities and routines. These preferences likely are based on the family's cultural orientation, learned practices, needs, and resources. For example, toy or object play may look different and have different importance across households, depending on a family's cultural practices and resources. Some families may have lots of purchased toys; others may creatively make toys out of common objects in their home (e.g., think about the many uses of paper, cardboard, plastic containers). Some households may emphasize toy or object play, whereas others emphasize books or quiet time.

One of the strengths of TGI and PoWRRS-Connect lies in their ability to work for a range of families, regardless of their cultural or socio-economic context. TGI requires no background knowledge about child development or communication from the family, only an appreciation of interacting. It requires no special resources to be successful and relies on no single routine or activity as the context for the implementation of PoWRRS-Connect. The only thing TGI requires of a family is that one caregiver be present and open to the possibilities of learning new ways to engage and communicate with the child. Believing in the importance of engagement and communication during the first year of life is critical. Savvy practitioners will use their training in birth-to-three service delivery to be responsive to the different strengths, needs, and priorities among families from a range of backgrounds.

ESTABLISHING AND MAINTAINING CHILD ENGAGEMENT

Establishing and maintaining child engagement throughout the PoWRRS-Connect cycle is critical both to support child learning and to help families feel successful in implementing the PoWRRS-Connect elements. The following sections offer tips for setting up clear opportunities, maximizing a child's visual skills, and making the most of toys and other objects. Presenting clear opportunities for communication provides a context for the child to begin to exert their independence within an exchange. Tips for creating engaging opportunities are presented. Because these opportunities often require shared visual attention on toys or other objects and rely on the child's visual response (via gaze with or without gestures and vocalizations), tips for maximizing a child's visual skills are offered. Strategies for working with children who have low vision or cortical visual impairment, or for whom visual abilities are unclear and/or inconsistent, are reviewed. Finally, the special role that toys play in providing experiences for children with moderate to severe physical disabilities is acknowledged, alongside ideas for making the most of toys and other objects when toys are not readily available in a child's environment. We hope that the videos offered throughout the book will help illustrate many of the ideas in this section.

Setting Up Clear Communication Opportunities

The PoWRRS-Connect cycle begins and ends with engagement through the connect element. Within these moments of connection between adult and child, the protocol is designed to offer a clear and salient opportunity for the child to become an active participant in the communicative exchange. Establishing and maintaining engagement with a communication partner may be easier for some children than others. Some children will respond to the presentation of an opportunity quickly. For example, a child may readily look, reach, and/or vocalize in response to just a brief pause from their communication partner. These are the children who have been waiting for the moment to show their independence and likely have a repertoire of untapped skills to do so. Other children may be equally motivated but may require more time to generate a response. Others still may be unaware that the opportunity to take a turn in a communicative exchange has been offered and thus remain passive throughout the interaction. The purpose of the providing opportunity (Po) element in PoWRRS-Connect is to pass the volley to the child. Opportunities offer a chance for the child to practice, with support, effecting control over their world. The mechanics of providing a communication opportunity are described in great detail in Chapter 6. Here, we discuss some of the subtler nuances.

When first modeling and then supporting caregivers in providing clear, salient, and well-paced opportunities, the practitioner should emphasize positioning. The adult's position relative to the child and, when using toys or other objects, the placement of those items can make or break a good opportunity. (Chapter 7 offered some specific advice regarding positioning for children with motor impairments.) In an ideal situation, the practitioner or caregiver will be at eye level with the child and within approximately 10–12 inches of the child's face. The adult should hold items just outside of the child's reach but in the child's line of vision. For maximum engagement, always make sure the child is attending to the objects being presented. For choice opportunities, objects should be at least 10 inches apart.

This presentation is ideal, but it may need to be modified depending on each child's abilities, interests, and motivations. For example, some children orient to objects better when they are first presented at midline and then slowly moved to 10 inches apart. Some children need to focus on one object for a bit of time, then the second item. This may require some trial and error as the practitioner and caregiver learn about the best presentation style for the child. The practitioner and caregiver also may experiment with the orientation of the toys or other objects presented. For example, the practitioner may first hold objects vertically but also explore presentation of objects horizontally. Chapter 6 and Appendix C provide videos that will illustrate the variety of ways to set up clear opportunities.

To maintain engagement throughout the opportunity, the practitioner or caregiver can manipulate visual cues such as exaggerated facial expressions or raised eyebrows, and auditory cues such as raising tone of voice or altering pitch, to elicit and maintain the child's engagement. Some children will benefit from exaggerating or turning up the volume on these cues to maximize their engagement whereas others will respond to softening or turning down the volume on these cues.

Maximizing Vision

Children with CCN will present with a range of visual abilities. Some may have intact visual acuity and visual processing skills, whereas others may have low vision, cortical visual impairment (CVI), or unknown or inconsistent visual skills. To benefit from TGI, all children should demonstrate a baseline ability to visually attend to either people or objects. Beyond this skill, it may be difficult to know the true visual capabilities of a young child with a complex profile. If concerns arise regarding a child's visual acuity or visual processing skills, the practitioner should consult with a vision specialist whenever possible. A vision specialist can provide a thorough assessment of the child's visual system and make specific recommendations to maximize the child's functional vision.

Many children with CCN (e.g., cerebral palsy, autism, Rett syndrome) experience CVI. CVI describes visual impairment caused by damage to the visual pathways that support visual processing in the brain (Roman-Lantzy, 2018). Because CVI is a brain-based visual impairment, many children often have healthy eyes but have trouble making meaning out of what they see. Although it is beyond the scope of this book to provide a comprehensive overview of CVI, some strategies that benefit children with CVI are included here to help practitioners and families maximize a child's vision and engagement. Practitioners may find these tips useful for any child with cognitive and/or motor challenges, whose visual skills and abilities are unclear or difficult to assess. We offer these ideas to help the practitioner and family in supporting the child in using their eyes for engagement and communication while awaiting further input from a vision specialist.

Children with visual processing difficulties can be overstimulated by visual information. Special attention should be paid to the properties of toys and other objects (see section on toys for further details) to maximize engagement rather than overwhelm. For example, it may be useful to avoid toys or items with multiple colors or complex patterns. Some children may have specific color preferences; introducing toys or other items that reflect these preferences may support sustained engagement during an interaction. Practitioners should carefully consider the size, spacing, and number of objects presented to a child. Many children cannot differentiate among very small objects, objects that are closely spaced together, or too many choices offered simultaneously. Looking away from choices that are presented can indicate to the practitioner or caregiver that the child is becoming overwhelmed. In these moments, practitioners or caregivers should simplify the interaction: use objects that are well defined against a solid background clear of visual clutter; space objects apart so that they may be easily differentiated; experiment with moving slowly when presenting one object and then another, allowing the child to attend to each; and keep things predictable. When the child knows what to expect and the pacing matches the child's processing, engagement likely will improve.

Finally, children with visual processing challenges like CVI may be sensitive to light in different ways. Some will benefit from backlighting objects (e.g., using a flashlight to draw the child's visual attention to an object or a communication partner's face) or using objects that have some light-up component to attract the child's visual attention. Other children may be distracted by light, such that the light itself becomes the most interesting thing in the room. A child who is unable to shift their gaze away from light may be signaling that the light is too stimulating and interfering with their ability to engage in the other rich components of the interaction.

We offer these tips for tailoring the interaction to maximize a child's visual abilities as broad suggestions. Many of these strategies require trial and error when working with a child and their family. We strongly encourage practitioners to consult with a vision specialist trained in the diagnosis and management of CVI if it is suspected that a child is not making progress due to compromised visual processing.

Making the Most of Toys and Their Properties

As suggested previously, toys, or everyday objects that can be used as toys, have a myriad of properties that should be considered as potential facilitators or barriers to eliciting and maintaining a child's engagement. Toys have visual properties (lights, colors), auditory characteristics (electronic or acoustic sounds, silence), tactile features (textures), and spatial qualities (round/curved, edges/corners). Each of these qualities can be used to support a child's engagement, but the practitioner must understand what a child likes or positively responds and what the child protests or turns away from. Also important to consider are the types of play opportunities a toy or object affords. Some toys are simple and offer opportunities to explore their visual, auditory, tactile, and/or spatial properties. Others afford the opportunity to explore and experience relationships between objects (e.g., putting things in/taking things out, connecting parts to a whole). Finally, toys and other objects also may support a child in moving from early exploratory to more advanced, functional play.

Although families differ in their views of toy play, play of any type is about engagement. Engagement between people and objects in their environment provides a ripe context for communication. As families differ, so do children's abilities to participate in play, particularly regarding play with toys and people. Children with CCN, especially those with significant motor impairments, often have reduced opportunities to independently explore objects or toys and experience the breadth of information that these objects provide as children begin to make sense of the world and their ability to act on and within it. For these children, play with toys may be extremely limited due to motor or cognitive disabilities, and because of these challenges, families might find toy play difficult.

Consider a child who is having difficulty grasping or manipulating toys or objects; in turn, the child or his family may not know how to play with toys in creative or nontraditional ways. Even with such variations among children and families, TGI has always recognized the value of toy play as a way to encourage engagement and communication. Practitioners can give families advice about types of toys to use, including suggesting adaptive toys that might be appropriate to match their children's unique needs. Practitioners can also model how to use toys, for example, hand-over-hand techniques that can be fun and stimulating for some children. Overall, TGI offers the opportunity for practitioners and families to work together to find ways to bring toy or object play into their routines, which can help build motor and cognitive skills such as object and object relation knowledge (i.e., causality) alongside communication and engagement. Play offers a crucial activity for children's learning about their world and how to share that learning with others.

> Play can be a natural and stimulating context for encouraging engagement and communication! However, remember play can look different from one family to the next depending on children's disabilities as well as families' resources and priorities.

The practitioner should carefully consider with the family what occasions the child has to explore and act on objects and the range of experiences the objects provide. Some children will readily reach out and engage with objects. Others will require a significant amount of physical support, including hand-over-hand assistance, to explore and play. Regardless of the level of support required, all children should be provided the opportunity to explore the objects in their world. The practitioner can emphasize to families the important role of object exploration and play for all children, as described previously, and support families to leverage toys and other objects for facilitating engagement throughout the PoWRRS-Connect cycle.

Finally, toys, or everyday objects used as toys, can be leveraged to elicit and sustain a child's engagement, thus extending an interaction and providing opportunities for the child to practice their communication skills. Although toys have a special role in supporting engagement, toys in the traditional sense are not required to successfully implement TGI through PoWRRS-Connect. Indeed, some families will not have access to toys in their home. As most practitioners know, simple household objects can be transformed into toys with just a little creativity and imagination. The recycling bin is a treasure box and should not be overlooked!

CONSIDERING VARIABILITY IN CHILDREN'S SKILLS AND ABILITIES

In previous chapters, we introduced children, through video exemplars and written vignettes, whose skills and abilities lie in different places along the continuum of communication behaviors. These children are meant to represent the variety of children a practitioner likely may encounter on their caseload. The Checklist of Early Communication Behaviors provided in this book serves as a resource for practitioners to evaluate children's skills and abilities along a proposed continuum of communication behaviors that is grounded in development. But what happens when children do not fit neatly on the continuum? The practitioner has the difficult job of being responsive to this variability and tailoring the PoWRRS-Connect elements to meet the individual needs of children and families, including those who do not neatly follow the proposed progression of conventional communication behaviors.

Children with moderate to severe disabilities and CCN are just that—complex! It can be difficult to determine their cognitive and communication abilities, especially when motor impairments affect performance. Some will not follow a linear path toward triadic gaze. Some children will use gestures, such as reaching without looking, more successfully than gaze. Some may get stuck in one place along the continuum and have difficulty moving forward. Some children may rely on their idiosyncratic behaviors. As the practitioner works with families and children, the practitioner will learn about the child's individual profile of skills. The practitioner should be vigilant about not extinguishing a child's preferred mode of communication simply because it does not fit along the proposed continuum. The communication continuum is meant to guide the practitioner based on what is known in the extant literature about how children typically progress through stages of early communication development. However, we do not know with certainty that all children will progress through the continuum as proposed. Chapter 9 describes ways to monitor children's progress through the continuum and offers ways of interpreting performance for adapting the supports provided.

TAILORING SHAPING

Shaping communication behaviors is often described as the "art" of the interaction and is often one of the most difficult elements of the PoWRRS-Connect protocol to implement for practitioners and caregivers. Shaping describes the prompts (verbal, visual, auditory, and tactile) that adults deliver in order to help a child produce a more sophisticated signal. This PoWRRS-Connect element has been described in detail in Chapter 6. The following discussion focuses on considerations for supporting caregivers in shaping their children's signals. During each interaction, the practitioner should carefully consider the types of prompts used, timing of delivery, and number of prompts delivered. Note that both the practitioner and the caregiver should be open to adjusting their approach so that the child has the opportunity to show what they know. Shaping is indeed an art and requires that adults be flexible and reflective about their role in supporting the child and understanding which shaping prompts best suit the child.

Prompt Selection

Sometimes practitioners rely on a standard set of prompts without realizing that their personal preferences or styles are driving the interaction. For example, it is easy to give verbal prompts (e.g., "look at me"), and they sometimes become the default. This tactic may lead to overlooking the benefits of other types of prompts. Sometimes the match between the practitioner or caregiver's preferences and the child's response is a good fit, but sometimes it is not. It is important to attend to how the child is responding to different types of prompts delivered by the adult. For example, an adult might find the tactile prompt of touching the child's face a useful way of getting the child's attention, but the child might not appreciate being touched. Paying attention to what prompts are given and how the child is responding takes conscious effort on the part of the practitioner or caregiver. Some reflective questions can be posed to help with this process: Does one modality of shaping (verbal, visual, auditory, tactile) seem to elicit a desired signal from the child more effectively or efficiently than others? Does the child get overwhelmed when multiple prompts are delivered all at once? Does the child benefit from shaping prompts used in combination with one another? Is there a "typical" set of shaping prompts that the practitioner or caregiver seems to rely on during each interaction? Are shaping prompts being faded over time?

Timing of Prompts

The practitioner should help caregivers consider when to prompt and, more importantly, when not to prompt the child to produce a more sophisticated signal. It is not appropriate (or even advisable) to shape every signal the child produces to triadic gaze. Shaping every behavior to a more conventional, sophisticated one can become frustrating for the child (and the caregiver). Practitioners should encourage caregivers to focus first on maintaining the child's engagement in the interaction and then on prompting more sophisticated behaviors. Above all, caregivers should be themselves and not feel as though they have to become teachers.

Amount of Prompting

At first, the child may require a lot of prompts to produce more conventional, sophisticated behaviors. That's fine! As the child practices expanding their repertoire of signals and experiences the reward of connection and engagement that results, the amount of prompting that is required should decrease over time. As the child demonstrates greater ease or increased frequency of production for a given target behavior, the adult should gradually fade prompts. The adult's goal is to help the child clearly request and choose, providing help as needed, but also fading prompts so the child will ultimately perform without assistance.

CONCLUSION

This chapter provided tips for tailoring TGI, focusing on four areas found to be important to making the PoWRRS-Connect protocol work for families: 1) making PoWRRS-Connect a natural part of caregiver–child interactions, 2) establishing and maintaining child engagement throughout the PoWRRS-Connect cycle, 3) considering variability in child skills and abilities, and 4) tailoring shaping to meet the needs of individual children. Table 8.2 provides a summary of these tips. The success in implementing PoWRRS-Connect will rely on the practitioner's ability to appropriately serve families. Recognizing how families typically interact with their children and appreciating what appears to be easy and hard about adopting PoWRRS-Connect will guide practitioners in their approach. Determining what families need will help practitioners figure out what to do (Gates, 2019).

The children and families for whom TGI is appropriate have complex needs. The tips offered in this chapter for tailoring the PoWRRS-Connect strategies are intended to support families in experiencing the joy of engaging with their children and to support children in reaching their fullest communicative potential. The journey that families and practitioners embark on through early support services often is just the beginning of unlocking this potential.

Table 8.2. Summary of tips for tailoring Triadic Gaze Intervention and PoWRRS-Connect

Making PoWRRS-Connect a natural part of caregiver–child interactions

Embed communication opportunities into authentic routines throughout the day.
- Understand and delineate the family's daily schedule of routines and activities.
- Recognize the little moments that arise within these routines and activities that present opportunities to focus on communication and engagement.
- Make PoWRRS-Connect a part of what is already occurring within a family's day; do not assign extra work.
- Refer to Table 8.1 as a starting point for ideas.

Support caregiver confidence and competence.
- Recognize and reinforce how the family is already supporting the child's engagement and communication (presume competence).
- Highlight the positive experiences between the caregiver and child; no successful moment of engagement is too small.
- Emphasize the connect element of PoWRRS-Connect.

Acknowledge and respect variation across families.
- Understand the individual family dynamics, including who assumes the role of primary caregiver and who makes decisions within the family unit.
- Recognize the different interaction styles and conventions present among caregiver–child dyads.
- Identify family priorities, needs, and resources.
- Discuss the family's preferences for routines and activities.
- Acknowledge and respect that these preferences and needs relate to their cultural orientation and learned paradigms.
- Incorporate families' cultural beliefs and practices into delivery of PoWRRS-Connect.

Establishing and maintaining child engagement

Set up clear communication opportunities.
- Present clear, salient, and well-paced opportunities.
- Make sure positioning between the adult and child is appropriate.
- Ensure placement of toys or objects is easy to see and access for the child.
- Pay attention to timing: Some children need more time than others.

Maximize vision
- Ensure that children can attend to people or objects.
- Pay attention to vision, and consider the possibility of cortical vision impairment.
- Consult with a vision specialist if concerns arise.
- Consider the properties of toys and other objects (e.g., color, shape, patterns) that may facilitate or impede a child's use of his other visual processing skills.
- Move slowly and reduce background visual clutter.
- Consider the role of backlighting.

Make the most of toys and other objects.
- Identify the visual, auditory, tactile, and spatial properties of objects that may be of interest to the child.
- Note the child's likes and dislikes as different objects are offered.
- Consider the opportunities afforded by different types of toys (e.g., spatial relationships between objects, functional actions on objects).
- Provide physical assistance to explore and engage with objects when appropriate or necessary.
- Expand the definition of toys to include any common household object that may elicit and hold a child's interest.

Considering variability in children's skills and abilities

- Recognize how a child fits onto the continuum of communication behaviors.
- Respond to less sophisticated behaviors first so that those behaviors become stabilized.
- Do not rush through the continuum; allow the child to practice less sophisticated behaviors—sometimes the child will need to spend more time on single focus behaviors (for example) before dual focus can be targeted.
- Appreciate that some children will not follow a linear path toward triadic gaze.

Tailoring shaping

Type of prompts
- Experiment with a variety of prompts, and note which are successful for the child.
- Pay attention to caregiver and child preferences—sometimes preferences align, and sometimes they do not; adjust prompts accordingly.

Timing of prompts
- Do not feel compelled to shape every behavior the child produces; focus on engagement first.
- Use judgment for when to push for more conventional, sophisticated behaviors.

Amount of prompts
- Use as many prompts as needed to elicit a target behavior at first, and then gradually fade over time.

CHAPTER 9

Monitoring Progress

Monitoring progress in EI is important for ensuring accountability and effective service delivery as practitioners work toward addressing family needs. Understanding the ways in which progress can be measured requires appreciation of several factors: EI service delivery system, the individual children, and children's families. Early intervention is a journey caregivers and practitioners travel together as they plan goals and share ideas for reaching them. For children with moderate to severe disabilities and CCN, the journey can feel slow because change can be gradual. In turn, monitoring change can be difficult because no one procedure can capture all the various and subtle ways children and families grow during their EI journey. Caregivers and practitioners will rely on each other to observe children's performances during daily routines so that when they meet with each other and with the EI team, they can discuss progress for two purposes: 1) tailoring and improving ongoing treatment, and 2) planning for the future.

Different states, agencies, and practitioners will have their own procedures for measuring progress during and after intervention, including number and spacing of visits for monitoring progress, methods for documenting change, and required reports. The commonality across these variations is monitoring change related to IFSP goals. Measuring progress on IFSP goals is critical, but because goals are typically broad, sometimes these data cannot capture the subtle, incremental changes that are occurring with some children with moderate to severe disabilities. This can be frustrating for the practitioner and the caregiver. This chapter offers ideas for monitoring behaviors directly related to engagement and communication to provide a more complete picture of children's progress. To be specific, observations of preverbal behaviors (e.g., gaze, gestures, vocalizations) and engagement in play with adults are recommended. This focus offers a window into the details that contribute to change in the IFSP goals. Observing progress in TGI-related areas may prove helpful for caregivers and practitioners in appreciating smaller changes for some children. Furthermore, the information should help in considering ways to improve current treatment and plan for the future.

The chapter begins with a general discussion of monitoring progress through IFSP goals. The value of data related directly to IFSP goals is highlighted, along with some of the limitations connected to relying only on IFSP outcomes for progress monitoring. The chapter then turns to describing ways to characterize progress by monitoring children's performance during activities involving communication and engagement from the perspective of TGI. This discussion offers suggestions for monitoring progress in two specific areas using the Checklist of Early Communication Behaviors ("Checklist") described initially in Chapter 5: 1) child production of preverbal communication behaviors (gaze, gestures, vocalizations), including sophistication, consistency, and independence of productions;

and 2) child toy or object play with others. The chapter describes each of the two areas and identifies specific behaviors that could be observed to reflect a child's learning and change over time. Data obtained about a child's performance in each of these areas can be easily recorded on the Checklist. The information obtained from making these observations is meant to capture small changes contributing to social engagement and communication that might be missed by focusing on only the broader IFSP outcomes. Will this be additional work for the practitioner? A little, but it will be well worth it. The recommended observations should blend easily with efforts to monitor IFSP goals. Simply put, the benefits of getting a more detailed look at children's progress will more than match the effort. The detailed information can be of great value for families of children with moderate to severe disabilities and CCN, whose development may be subtle, slow, and difficult to document. Completing the Checklist at the initial assessment, during service delivery, and at the annual review can provide a truly helpful visual aid to share with families. This more comprehensive view of a child's achievements can give caregivers a better understanding of their children's abilities and will assist the caregiver and practitioner in working together to plan ongoing and future intervention.

Figure 9.1 illustrates the conceptual framework described in this chapter to monitor children's progress. At the top of the figure is the IFSP goal that drives procedures for measuring progress. Below the IFSP goal are the two TGI areas related to IFSP goals: child production of conventional, preverbal communication behaviors and child toy or object play with others. Information gathered from the IFSP goal measurement and observations of children's communication behaviors and toy or object play come together to inform how the caregiver and practitioner think about intervention and the need to alter it and plan for the future.

MEASURING PROGRESS THROUGHOUT SERVICE DELIVERY

Monitoring progress is tied primarily to the IFSP as mandated by federal law. IFSP goals are written so that they specify child and family outcomes and procedures for measuring these outcomes. These procedures indicate where, when, and how the outcomes will be measured for each IFSP goal. The measurements typically occur at quarterly or semiannual intervals, with the practitioner and family noting changes that have occurred and discussing them with the birth-to-three team. Critical information from this discussion is documented in some type of staffing report. During the year, measured outcomes allow for revisiting the IFSP and revising goals and objectives as necessary. Annual measurement of the IFSP goals and achievements of progress are documented in a final report. In some cases, tests or other tools may be readministered. These measurement procedures provide important information for evaluating the success of the supports provided in regard to achieving IFSP goals. As a part of the final evaluation, progress on individual IFSP goals contributes to monitoring for the three major child outcomes of EI services delineated by the U.S. Office of Special Education Programs (OSEP) (ECTA, 2021; Office of Special Education Programs, 2019):

1. Children's demonstration of positive social relationships, as reflected by how well children relate to those around them.

2. Children's acquisition and use of knowledge and skills, as reflected by thinking, learning, reasoning, memory, and problem-solving skills.

3. Children's ability to take action for meeting their needs, as reflected by their being able to take care of themselves and/or use appropriate ways to have their needs met.

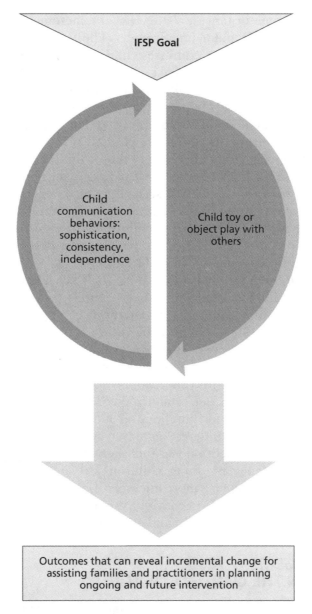

Child communication behaviors: sophistication, consistency, independence

Child toy or object play with others

IFSP Goal

Outcomes that can reveal incremental change for assisting families and practitioners in planning ongoing and future intervention

Figure 9.1. Monitoring progress: Individualized family service plan (IFSP) goals and areas related to Triadic Gaze Intervention for capturing change.

Progress on IFSP goals and the broader summary of outcomes listed previously appropriately capture success of early supports as they correspond to the federal mandates of providing services that address families' needs and are grounded in families' daily routines. In complying with these mandates, individual states, agencies, and birth-to-three teams design their own child and family outcomes and measurement procedures to obtain necessary data for addressing the IFSP goals and OSEP requirements, which in turn inform current and future planning for recommended services.

Monitoring IFSP goals is clearly valuable; however, for children with moderate to severe disabilities, gradual, subtle changes in progress might not be captured through IFSP monitoring alone. In some instances, change may be incremental and difficult to detect, particularly in children with motor impairments. These changes may not be revealed by the IFSP goal measurement, which addresses children's performance in broader domains of functioning, as indicated previously (e.g., social relationships, problem solving, meeting daily needs). This population of children by definition experience challenges in their development and may experience further compromises from ongoing medical issues. Their performances may be difficult to discern or interpret. For example, a child's motor involvement might mask clear efforts to act on people and objects in the environment. Their performances might appear simple because of motor limitations and thus do not appear conventional (e.g., a slight body lean vs. a clear arm extension and point). In addition, the children's performances are often described as inconsistent, influenced by a variety of factors, both internal (e.g., periodic, fleeting seizures) and external (e.g., routines with favorite toys vs. those without). Overall, the children may rely on adult support in the form of prompts to demonstrate their best performances. The developmental and physiological challenges facing this population of children may make measuring progress difficult in the confines of the IFSP. This is because IFSP goals are inherently broad because they are written to reflect functional outcomes tied to family routines. This is not to say that practitioners and caregivers cannot observe nuanced changes within IFSP measurement procedures but rather that doing so may be hard.

This chapter gives practitioners suggestions for easily observing and documenting small changes in engagement and communication through the lens of TGI. The focus of TGI allows for drilling down into the details of broader IFSP goals by looking more explicitly at particular aspects of performance during routine activities. The information obtained can serve to highlight for families and support teams the children's competencies, which might otherwise be underestimated or overlooked. So often, families, practitioners, and agencies struggle to document change in young children with severe disabilities. By observing on a more micro level, as suggested by monitoring TGI-related behaviors, valuable changes, even though small, can be seen and celebrated.

> When monitoring progress, consider children's incremental change!

MONITORING ENGAGEMENT AND COMMUNICATION IN THE CONTEXT OF TGI

As has been argued throughout this book, engagement and communication are foundational to development across domains. Furthermore, engagement and communication as targeted through TGI contribute to the major child outcomes associated with support services: increasing positive social relationships, acquiring and using skills, and taking action to meet one's needs. As such, monitoring progress of behaviors within the context of TGI can reveal valuable, detailed information for families, practitioners, and agencies about changes achieved through providing early supports. To be specific, two areas of TGI can be easily observed and monitored using the Checklist: 1) child production of conventional preverbal communication behaviors (gaze, gestures, vocalizations), specifically, sophistication, consistency, and independence of productions; and 2) child toy or object play with others. The recommendation is that these two areas be examined in the context of appropriate IFSP goals. However, sometimes, to get the most accurate picture of a child's progress, the two areas should be examined during a variety of family routines. The type of observations to be made are described next, as well as illustrations of how data can be easily recorded on the Checklist. (*Note:* The Checklist is available in Appendix B for duplication; it is also available as a resource on the Brookes Download Hub along with the other downloadable resources for this book.) The practitioner should collect the kinds of data that are easiest and most informative, either enumerating observations or writing anecdotal notes. Examples of these kinds of data are discussed next. The assumption is that observation of engagement and communication can be made during any visit, but to complement measurement of IFSP goals, these observations with data collection should be made when required by individual agencies (i.e., quarterly, semiannually, or annually). The discussion that follows describes what should be observed in the two areas and why the data would be informative for documenting change that complements the IFSP goal measurements. Following the discussion, an example of monitoring progress for a specific child is provided to illustrate observation and data collection using the Checklist and how the data might be interpreted.

Monitoring Progress by Observing Children's Communication Behaviors

TGI has used the continuum of communication behaviors, delineated in the Checklist introduced in Chapter 5, to describe the development of engagement and preverbal communication. The Checklist defines the well-documented conventional gaze, gestural, and vocal behaviors that develop over time from pre-intentional to intentional forms of communication prior to first words. This continuum reflects the incremental changes that can occur during the first year of life as children learn to participate in social relationships and navigate their world to accomplish their wants and needs. Using this framework, the Checklist provides a practical tool that practitioners can use to document children's acquisition and use of gaze, gestural, and vocal behaviors over time during everyday activities. Logically, then, the Checklist can also be utilized for monitoring progress of communication as part of engaged interactions along with measurement of the IFSP goals. The discussion that follows will focus on the production of preverbal communication behaviors and explore the details about how children with moderate to severe disabilities and CCN might acquire these behaviors incrementally over time through receiving early supports. Acquisition of preverbal behaviors comprising engagement and communication are examined from three perspectives:

1. Sophistication of productions (simple to complex)

2. Consistency of productions (inconsistent to consistent)

3. Independence of productions (dependent on support to independent)

Examining children's productions of behaviors from these three perspectives can provide a detailed reflection of progress as children gradually increase the clarity and control of behaviors when engaging and communicating with others. Figure 9.2 illustrates how increased sophistication, consistency, and independence of productions will, in turn, lead to increased clarity and control of efforts to engage and communicate.

Observing Sophistication in Production of Communication Behaviors Completing the Checklist based on caregiver report and practitioner observation provides a way to easily monitor the behaviors a child uses to engage with others and communicate their wants and needs during authentic routines. The Checklist allows for a straightforward way

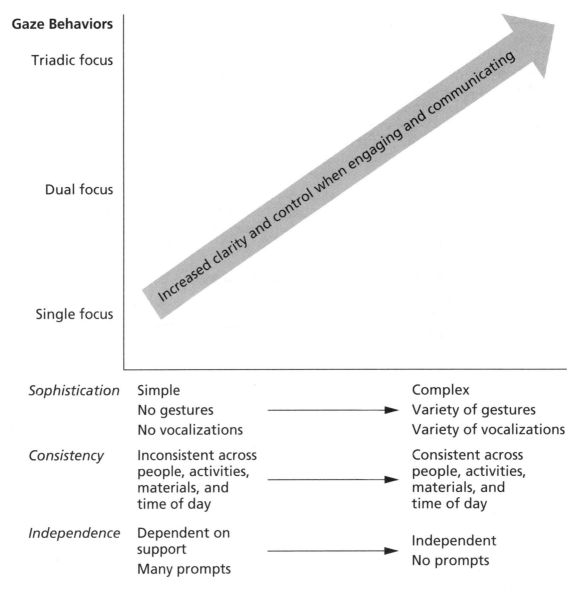

Figure 9.2. Monitoring changes in gaze, gestures, and vocalizations to reveal increased clarity and control in engagement and communication.

to document early emerging gaze behaviors along the continuum from pre-intentional to intentional (i.e., single to dual, to triadic focus). (See Chapter 5 to review instructions on completing the Checklist.) The practitioner can monitor not only this vertical/developmental dimension of progress but also the growing complexity in communication efforts as exhibited by children's production of more and varied gestures and vocalizations to accompany gaze behaviors. To be specific, the Checklist allows for recording particular gestures occurring with gaze, including leaning, reaching, pointing, showing, and giving. Vocalizations can also be specified on the Checklist, including simple consonant and vowel productions, to consonant–vowel combinations, to phonetically consistent forms that resemble early words. As a child develops along the continuum from single, to dual, to triadic focus, and increases variety of gestures and vocalization, the child's communication will become more sophisticated. Figure 9.2 illustrates the way communication behaviors may change, with eye gaze displayed vertically and increased variety of gestures and vocalizations displayed horizontally on the first line. As illustrated in the figure, as children acquire more sophisticated gaze, gestural, and vocal behaviors, they will gain clarity and control when engaging and communicating with others.

By completing the Checklist over time, practitioners and caregivers can track children's improving ability to produce gaze, gestures, and vocalizations, which might not be appreciated if the IFSP goal is the only measure of progress. The Checklist can be completed any time during intervention to document change of behaviors that contribute to clarity and increased control during engagement and communication. The use of these data will not only inform progress but will allow practitioners and caregivers to work together as they evaluate and modify their implementation of PoWRRS-Connect. For example, at a quarterly measurement session, the caregiver might note that her child has started reaching and vocalizing when requesting more during snack time. The practitioner and caregiver might decide to encourage this behavior along with looking at her mother during the next phase of services. This type of nuanced change might not have been readily captured during a quarterly IFSP goal measurement, which might only capture the child's continuing need to work on the goal. Likewise, the child's gaze, gestures, and vocalizations should also be monitored annually. The status of the child's behaviors at this time will be critical for determining future directions for the child's skill development in communication, including consideration of whether to introduce alternative and augmentative supports to the child's plan. To illustrate, consider a child who is producing triadic gaze and using a variety of vocalizations and phonetically consistent forms that are increasingly close to words at the annual evaluation. The practitioner and caregiver might use this information as a basis for discussing the child's possible benefit from intervention that focuses on spoken word productions. For a child who is not producing any type of vocalization, but rather relying on gaze and gestures, some form of alternative and augmentative support might be introduced. Thus, monitoring progress on the production of gaze, gestural, and vocal behaviors using the Checklist can be extremely helpful for tailoring services to match children's strengths and needs and as a way to provide more detail to the IFSP measurement.

Observing Consistency in Production of Communication Behaviors   The Checklist's breakdown of behaviors allows for observation of not only specific behaviors that demonstrate increased sophistication of performance, but also consistency across contexts and time as well. By examining performance during a variety of routines (including different activities, materials, and partners), practitioners and caregivers can monitor a child's stability in the production of behaviors over time. This stability contributes to the child's increased clarity and control of behaviors when engaging and communicating with others. Figure 9.2 illustrates developing consistency in the production of communication behaviors along the horizontal axis.

As an example, some children's learning may be tied to particular people or objects at the beginning of intervention but will gradually expand to other people and objects over time. Another change in consistency might be captured in how children use new behaviors; that is, some children might perform differently depending on the purpose of the communication. For example, some children might produce particular communication behaviors only when requesting, but over time they will expand their productions to commenting. Time of day can also influence consistency of performance. For example, some children may be less vocal as they approach naptime. These variations are important to document for appreciating consistency and improvement in performance and may not be captured by the IFSP goal measurement. The Checklist has a column for notes where practitioners can enter key information about people, activities, materials, and time of day during the interaction. As practitioners investigate progress, part of their responsibility is analyzing inconsistencies in performance and sharing them with the support team; inconsistencies for children with CCN can indicate problems with the treatment approach or could reveal something going on with the child (e.g., health). The information described may prove helpful to practitioners and caregivers as they seek to identify factors contributing to consistency in performance, which can inform recommendations in the short term and the future.

Observing Independence in Production of Communication Behaviors

Related to monitoring sophistication and consistency in the production of early communication behaviors is recognizing the degree to which a child's performance needs to be supported by adult assistance. When monitoring progress, the practitioner should pay attention to which communication behaviors can be produced with and without prompts from the adult.

Why is this important? Imagine these different scenarios concerning a child's performance with and without assistance. Consider a child who may consistently produce dual focus with gestures with considerable prompting by an adult, but when those prompts are removed, the child's level of performance declines to a different behavior, single focus. This child does not yet have control over dual focus. Consider another child who can consistently produce dual focus with no prompts and can only inconsistently produce triadic focus with considerable prompting. This child would be said to have control of dual focus and is learning triadic focus. Therefore, when monitoring a child's progress, it might be helpful to track the type and amount of prompting required for shedding light on how independent a child's performance becomes over time. Monitoring progress from the perspective of needed support allows a look at the process of learning new skills. This perspective might capture a child's performance of a particular behavior as it moves from highly supported to independent over the course of birth-to-three services. This change would provide evidence of a child's mastery of a skill. A child's ability to produce a behavior or solve a problem without help from others reflects their learning and acquisition of an ability that will generate additional learning. Figure 9.2 illustrates how independence in performance (along the horizontal axis) can contribute to improved engagement and communication. As children become less dependent on adult assistance in their productions, they will be able to increase their clarity and control of behaviors and more successfully engage and communicate with others.

The Checklist can be useful for gathering information about growing independence in performance over time. Because different behaviors are observed during a monitoring session, comments can be added to the Checklist regarding type and amount of prompting that was used by the adult. In an ideal situation, the Checklist would show a decrease in adult assistance and an increase in child independence. Table 9.1 highlights the kinds of data that might be recorded on the Checklist regarding adult prompts and child performance. The reader will recognize the type of prompts from Chapters 5, 6, and 8. When tracking

Table 9.1. Observing children's need for support during engagement and communication: Types and amount of prompting

	Observing support
Types of prompts	Verbal
	Visual
	Auditory
	Tactile
Amount of prompting	Maximum assistance (e.g., several types offered together and repeated)
	Moderate assistance (e.g., one type and repeated)
	Minimal assistance (e.g., one type)
	No assistance (e.g., child produces behavior independently and repeatedly)

prompts for monitoring progress, practitioners can choose to quantify this information or note it anecdotally in the Checklist. In either case, the data can be useful for monitoring change that might not otherwise be observed. Furthermore, the information can also help the practitioner and caregiver appreciate the types and amounts of prompting that seem most useful for a child, which will help plan for intervention in the short term and the future.

Monitoring Progress by Observing Children's Toy or Object Play With Others

In addition to examining children's early preverbal gaze, gestural, and vocal behaviors, other aspects of engagement and communication related to TGI offer an opportunity to monitor progress. *Remember:* TGI's focus on engagement and communication also contributes to facilitating early cognitive development, particularly knowledge of people and objects and relationships between them. The implementation of PoWRRS-Connect across all types of routines during a child's and family's day, including play, will stimulate all kinds of development. When we have talked about play, we have included both social play (e.g., Peekaboo) and play with toys or objects (e.g., blocks, plastic containers). Specifically examining a child's development of toy or object play with others over time offers another way of observing nuanced developmental changes. When deciding to observe toy or object play as a way to monitor progress, individual families and practitioners should discuss and weigh the value in doing so given the families' beliefs and priorities. As discussed in Chapter 8, play can mean different things to different families, and the suggestions for using it as a way to monitor progress should be filtered through this lens. Engagement with others around a shared toy or object can provide a unique opportunity to examine progress in development. Over the years, the outcomes of TGI have demonstrated that not only do children's engagement with others and communicative behaviors change, but so does the quantity and quality of their play. To be specific, toy play is an activity that naturally brings families and children together: exploring, communicating, and enjoying each other's company. This context provides an exciting learning environment and, as such, an avenue for observing and monitoring change.

The TGI research has demonstrated this unique role of toy or object play, even for children with severe motor impairments. Following participation in TGI, children spent more time exploring and manipulating toys during play. Children moved from early developing play behaviors, such as mouthing or shaking, to moving individual parts of toys, to exploring cause–effect actions and for some children using toys functionally. Also, over time, children appeared to gradually play with a greater variety of toys, moving from simple toys (e.g., textured objects), to toys with parts and functional toys (e.g., toy brush, cup). Note that children's solicitation of adult involvement during play increased as well; the children were observed literally reaching out to the adults to make them part of their play routines. These findings have been observed by practitioners as well as reported by caregivers (Feuerstein et al., 2018; Olswang & Pinder, 1995). Caregivers also anecdotally noted their enjoyment dur-

> A parent's comments on the power of purposeful play: "I really believe her [the practitioner's] play with B gave him a sense of control over his environment. I learned that all children have essentially the same needs: to play, to learn. Our son wanted to play. He was actually interested in toys for the first time, and he wanted to share his discoveries with me"
>
> (Olswang & Pinder, 1995).

ing toy play increased over time, perhaps because they could more readily recognize their children's communicative attempts, which enhanced their engagement. Thus, observing caregiver–child interactions specifically during toy play can be a valuable addition to other outcomes for monitoring progress.

Based on this research and years of implementing TGI, caregivers and practitioners are encouraged to use the context of play with toys for observing not only engagement and communication but also children's actual play, including types of toys selected by the child and how they are manipulated. Table 9.2 highlights observation categories for toy or object play that emerged in the research described previously and might be valuable for monitoring progress (Olswang & Pinder, 1995). These aspects of play also can be easily documented in the notes section of the Checklist. Toy play, therefore, can supplement observation of child communication behaviors to provide a fuller picture

Table 9.2. Observing children's toy or object play with adults: Possible observation categories and examples

Observing toy or object play	
Observation categories	Examples
Type of toy	Squeeze toys
	Textured toys
	Toys with parts
	Toys that can be activated
	Functional toys
Type of play or manipulation	Mouthing
	Touching
	Shaking
	Banging
	Throwing
	Part relations (e.g., on and off, in and out, open and close)
	Exploring cause–effect action using the adult
	Using object functionally (e.g., combing hair)

Source: Olswang & Pinder (1995).

of the nature of a child's engagement and interactions with others. Practitioners can choose to quantify this information or note it anecdotally. In either case, the data can be useful for monitoring changes that might not otherwise be observed if only measuring the IFSP goals. Again, for some children who are developing slowly and showing incremental changes in birth-to-three services, toy play may offer valuable insight into their developmental progress.

EXAMPLE OF MONITORING PROGRESS IN THE CONTEXT OF TGI

In this section of the chapter, we return to Sophie, the child introduced in Chapter 5, to provide an example of data sampling the two areas of TGI that can be used to supplement the measurement of an IFSP goal. Each scenario provides a description of Sophie's progress and offers a completed Checklist to capture her communication behaviors and toy play at the time of the monitoring session. First, a scenario is presented to illustrate data collection for monitoring progress for the purpose of altering and improving Sophie's ongoing treatment. This scenario represents a semiannual review. Second, another scenario is presented to illustrate data collection for planning Sophie's future communication needs. This scenario represents the annual review. To get started, recall the following description of Sophie, the family's priority during initial assessment, the identified routine for focus, and Sophie's IFSP goal:

Sophie

Sophie is a 13-month-old girl with Down syndrome and associated moderate physical disabilities. Her muscle tone is flaccid (weak), and she requires support to sit. She is gaining trunk control. She has limited reaching and grasping. Her temperament is easygoing; she loves being around people. She primarily focuses on people; she seldom looks at objects without lots of encouragement from others.

Family's Priority

Sophie's parents explain, "We want Sophie to play with her older brother and sister. She adores both of them—they make her laugh and smile more than anyone else! But right now, she just watches them having fun; she's not really part of the action. She could just sit and watch them forever. We would love to see her actually participate or take a turn in their games."

Identified Routine and/or Activity

Sophie's siblings spend about 10 minutes playing together in the mornings, right before getting on the school bus. Mom is usually sitting with the children during this time while Dad packs up the kids' lunches. Sometimes the older kids will toss a ball back and forth outside as they wait for the bus to arrive or play with toys inside as they wait.

Possible IFSP Goal

During their morning play routine, Sophie will take a turn playing with toys with her brother and sister by looking at the toy and/or leaning forward to reach for it when one of her siblings holds it up and asks, "Do you want a turn?" three times across 5 days.

Two Scenarios to Illustrate Monitoring Progress

The two scenarios that follow focus specifically on examining Sophie's communication behaviors and her toy or object play during a semiannual and annual review for monitoring progress. Figures 9.4 and 9.5, respectively, illustrate Checklists that have been completed for the observations made during these reviews. In these scenarios, the mother and the primary service provider, an SLP, are working together to discuss and observe Sophie's progress. The mother reports on the morning routine with Sophie's brother and sister to provide information directly about the IFSP goal. In addition, the mother wants to show the SLP some of Sophie's skills, so she engages in other family routines during the visit. These other routines provide an opportunity to observe Sophie's consistency in performance, the need for adult prompting, and toy play in other contexts.

Scenario 1: 6-Month Semiannual Review   Recall that during the initial assessment, Sophie was able to shift her gaze from a communication partner to a shared object or toy during a play routine only when she was provided with prompts, such as shaking the toy. This ability to shift gaze from person to object (or object to person) is a building block toward triadic gaze production (the back-and-forth looking between object and adult with or without gestures and vocalizations). Figure 9.3 provides the completed Checklist reflecting this initial assessment performance. Given that Sophie was stimulable for moving her gaze from adults to objects but not yet producing this behavior independently, gaze shifts from people to objects was identified as an appropriate place to start employing TGI and PoWRRS-Connect. Sophie's family has been focusing on this behavior during routines throughout the day, and more specifically during activities that resembled the IFSP goal of taking turns playing with a ball and other toys with her brother and sister for the last 6 months. In this scenario, the focus is on the semiannual visit for monitoring progress.

Mom reported that Sophie was continuing to enjoy watching her siblings play ball before school but now seemed more engaged. She noted that Sophie is clearly looking at her brother and sister—and looking at the ball while reaching for it—which is being interpreted as a request to participate. She likes to try rolling the ball back and forth to them and has begun doing so with others, including Dad, Mom, and Grandma. Mom reported this has prompted the family to introduce a few new toys in the morning. During this visit, Sophie was also observed playing with a new toy, a busy box, with her mother and having juice and crackers during snack time. Figure 9.4 reflects the mother's report and the SLP's observations during this visit.

As illustrated in Figure 9.4, Sophie needs no assistance in producing single focus on objects and people, and she needs periodic assistance for dual focus (looking from object to person or person to object). The mother reported this, and the practitioner observed it during play and snack. When given a choice during snack, Sophie would primarily look at her choice and even fuss a bit; she needed a prompt to look at her mom. Mom reported that Sophie is making more sounds when she interacts with others. This was observed during the session, including increased production of vowels and consonants (though limited in quantity and variety), and a repeated consonant–vowel combination (*mu mu*), along with leaning and reaching. Both Mom and the SLP were pleased to see these communication behaviors, which Mom reported helped her better understand what Sophie was "saying." When Sophie was playing with the busy box and her mother, she was observed to be clearly engaged; she vocalized and tried to grossly manipulate the levers on the busy box. Sophie couldn't get the levers to work on her own and began to get frustrated. After waiting for about 15 seconds, Mom asked Sophie if she wanted help. The practitioner observed

Checklist of Early Communication Behaviors

Name: *Sophie (initial assessment)*

Foundational Behaviors for Triadic Gaze			Source of Information		Notes
			Caregiver Reported	Practitioner Observed	Activity or Routine, Toys or Objects, People Present, Prompts Used
Gaze	Single Focus	Looks and sustains gaze to a **person***	✔	✔	
		Looks and sustains gaze to an **object***	✔	✔	*Needed considerable prompting to look at toy (shaking toy)*
		Follows a moving **object***	✔	✔	*After getting her attention to toy*
	Dual Focus	Looks back and forth between **two objects***		✔	*During playtime on the floor with Mom: focused on one object at a time—not yet looking back and forth.*
		Looks from **object to person OR person to object***		✔	*Can't yet shift from a person to an object—gets "stuck." Will look at the object when provided a prompt—shaking the object.*
	Triadic Focus	Looks **back and forth** between object **AND** person*			
Vocalizations		Produces **early sounds** (fusses, squeals)		✔	*Open vowels only.*
		Produces **consonants, vowels, and consonant–vowel combinations**			
		Produces **word approximations**			
Gestures		**Leans/reaches** for object **OR** person*			
		Shows, points, gives			
		Uses **gestures** meaningfully (waves hi/bye, covers eyes for Peekaboo)			

*NOTE: Be sure to note if the child also uses vocalizations and/or gestures when looking.

Figure 9.3. Checklist of Early Communication Behaviors: Sophie's initial assessment.

Checklist of Early Communication Behaviors

Name: *Sophie (6-month semiannual review)*

Foundational Behaviors for Triadic Gaze			Source of Information		Notes
			Caregiver Reported	Practitioner Observed	Activity or Routine, Toys or Objects, People Present, Prompts Used
Gaze	Single Focus	Looks and sustains gaze to a **person***	✔	✔	*No adult prompts needed.*
		Looks and sustains gaze to an **object***	✔	✔	*Busy box—while manipulating levers.*
		Follows a moving **object***	✔	✔	*Ball play with siblings (mother report), snack*
	Dual Focus	Looks back and forth between **two objects***	✔	✔	*Snack and toy play given a choice. No adult prompts needed.*
		Looks from **object to person OR person to object***	✔	✔	*Ball play with sibling (mother report), busy box, snack, inconsistently needed a prompt during choice (during snack, she focused primarily on her preference and even fussed a bit).*
	Triadic Focus	Looks **back and forth** between object **AND** person*		✔	*Observed one time, when Sophie was indicating that she needed her mother's help with a toy. Sophie was slow in looking between her mom and the object; when her mother repeated, "Do you need my help pushing? I can help you open the box," a fleeting back and forth between object and mom occurred.*
Vocalizations		Produces **early sounds** (fusses, squeals)			
		Produces **consonants, vowels, and consonant–vowel combinations**	✔	✔	*Open vowels and some consonants Production of consonant–vowel combination (mu mu), repeated over and over while looking at Mother*
		Produces **word approximations**			
Gestures		**Leans/reaches** for object **OR** person*	✔	✔	*Leaning/reaching toward the busy box while vocalizing and looking between Mom and toy Also observed independently trying to manipulate levers on busy box and successfully doing so with hand-over-hand assistance from Mother*
		Shows, points, gives			
		Uses **gestures** meaningfully (waves hi/bye, covers eyes for Peekaboo)			

*NOTE: Be sure to note if the child also uses vocalizations and/or gestures when looking.

Figure 9.4. Checklist of Early Communication Behaviors: Sophie's 6-month semiannual review.

Sophie look between the object and mom, and then she gave a single fleeting look back at the object (i.e., triadic gaze). Sophie's response was acknowledged by hand-over-hand help from her mother in operating the toy.

This *6-month semiannual review* revealed that Sophie had made some important changes in communication and engagement. Visually these changes are easily seen by placing the Checklist completed at the initial assessment (Figure 9.3) next to the one completed at the semiannual review (Figure 9.4). As can be seen, Sophie made good progress in looking at objects versus looking only at the adult, as was observed during the initial assessment. She was also producing new vocalizations and gestures to accompany her eye gaze. Furthermore, Sophie seemed to have begun connecting people and objects, as she was looking between them with adequate waiting and few prompts; this was reported by her mother and observed by the SLP. Observing the one fleeting triadic focus when given a clear prompt by her mother was exciting. The SLP and mother talked about the importance of practice and stabilizing Sophie's behaviors. They discussed how to adapt the IFSP goal by emphasizing looking between objects and people and reinforcing this back-and-forth looking. The practitioner gave Sophie's mom ideas for how to support this signal and even how to try to shape a full triadic gaze. Mom thought she would feel most comfortable trying to build her back-and-forth looking during meal/snack time so that became the focus for the coming weeks. Along with building her gaze behaviors, plans were discussed for trying to encourage vocalizations and gestures. Mom was urged to model a variety of sounds but not require Sophie to produce them. Sophie's motor involvement might affect her efforts to form clear gestures and manipulate toys, so the SLP talked about ways to encourage participation given these challenges. The SLP discussed different types of toys and ways in which to encourage object exploration and operation. Mom was excited about Sophie's increased engagement and participation in all kinds of activities. She noted particularly that involving all the children in the morning routine was really successful and helpful to starting their day. She even thought that Sophie's siblings would be eager to expand the way they played with toys and encourage Sophie's looking.

Scenario 2: 12-Month Annual Review

In this scenario, the focus is on the annual visit for monitoring progress. The SLP visited the family, asked about Sophie's performance in various routines, and observed Sophie and her mother playing with blocks and a sorting box. Figure 9.5 provides a completed Checklist to illustrate Sophie's year-end accomplishments. As illustrated in Figure 9.5, Mom reported that Sophie was using her eyes to look at people and at objects a lot more. Mom reported and the practitioner observed that Sophie primarily used dual focus (looking at object and adult); when she did produce a fleeting triadic gaze, it was when she wanted help or was requesting more. Triadic gaze occurred when Sophie started by looking at the adult, then the object, and quickly to the adult again. It was limitedly observed when she started with the object. Furthermore, triadic gaze always needed a long wait by the adult plus a verbal prompt (e.g., "Don't forget to look at me," "Look at the X [pause]; now look back at me"). Auditory cues, such as shaking toys, or tapping them on the table was helpful in getting Sophie to look at the object as part of the gaze shift. She produced a triadic gaze with the SLP during a choice activity when considerable prompting was given.

Mom was happy to report that Sophie is doing some imitating, including some gestures and play (e.g., banging blocks together). Mom noted that the imitating was relatively new and that it was exciting to see because it really felt like a way to engage and take turns with Sophie in all kinds of activities. Sophie's grasp is coming along, which helps for more toy play. She is starting to show objects when prompted with a verbal cue. She tries to imitate when Mom models showing. Sophie continues to be a quiet child, only producing open CV

Checklist of Early Communication Behaviors

Name: *Sophie (12-month annual review)*

Foundational Behaviors for Triadic Gaze			Source of Information		Notes
			Caregiver Reported	Practitioner Observed	Activity or Routine, Toys or Objects, People Present, Prompts Used
Gaze	Single Focus	Looks and sustains gaze to a **person***	✔	✔	
		Looks and sustains gaze to an **object***	✔	✔	
		Follows a moving **object***	✔	✔	
	Dual Focus	Looks back and forth between **two objects***	✔	✔	
		Looks from **object to person OR person to object***	✔	✔	*Observed during request and choice and never as a "comment"*
	Triadic Focus	Looks **back and forth** between object **AND** person*		✔	*Produced during requests for help or more, always needing a long wait and a prompt, "Look at me," "Look at the X"* *Lots of prompting to get triadic gaze during a choice activity* *Mom noticed more attempts at gestures too along with gaze shifts (see below).*
Vocalizations		Produces **early sounds** (fusses, squeals)			
		Produces **consonants, vowels,** and **consonant–vowel combinations**	✔	✔	*Open vowels, limited consonants* *Consonant–vowel combination but limited variety* *Primarily mu mu. Quiet. Not imitating sounds*
		Produces **word approximations**			
Gestures		**Leans/reaches** for object **OR** person*	✔	✔	*Reaches and grasps objects* *Reaches are frequent with gaze shift as a way to ask for help.* *Sophie seems to be practicing this, as observed with the blocks and sorting box.*
		Shows, points, gives	✔	✔	*Tries to show when holding an object, when Mom asks, "What do you have; can you show me?" Most successful when Mom models and provides a little assistance. Observed trying to imitate.*
		Uses **gestures** meaningfully (waves hi/bye, covers eyes for Peekaboo)			*Tries to wave bye-bye when asked and a model is given* *More manipulating of toy parts* *Also trying to bang toys together when asked and a model is given*

*NOTE: Be sure to note if the child also uses vocalizations and/or gestures when looking.

Figure 9.5. Checklist of Early Communication Behaviors: Sophie's 12-month annual review.

syllables that sound like "more more." She is not imitating sounds. Given these end-of-year observations, the practitioner and mother talked about how far Sophie had progressed over the year and what might be next. A more solid dual focus and emerging triadic gaze and gestures, along with increased toy exploration and imitation, are wonderful accomplishments and open up many options for future goals.

For the next quarter, the practitioner and mother discussed the value of further encouraging triadic gaze as a way to actively engage with Sophie and offer a way that Sophie can exert control over her environment. The practitioner encouraged Mom to reinforce Sophie's efforts to produce this behavior not only in requesting "more" or "help," but also in choosing and even commenting where it seemed appropriate. For example, Mom could encourage gaze shifting when Sophie is enjoying a toy by saying, "Show it to Grandma." Mom and the practitioner discussed toy play, and Mom shared about Sophie's favorite types of play; this discussion included ways of further expanding some of the toy or object options that seemed appropriate. They discussed the value of encouraging more gestures, too. The practitioner showed Mom how to model different communication gestures. Sophie's motor involvement might interfere with gesture formation, so the practitioner helped give Mom ideas for some simple ones, such as "shaking her head no" when Sophie didn't want something. The practitioner encouraged modeling that did not require Sophie to imitate as a way of building skills that might lead to Sophie's possibly learning early signs. These ideas, along with others, would contribute to the discussion about new IFSP goals.

The value of observing and recording Sophie's performance of TGI-related behaviors at three time points (initial assessment, semiannual review, and annual review) offers a valuable examination of change. Viewing Figure 9.3 (Checklist for initial assessment) next to Figure 9.4 (Checklist for semiannual review) and Figure 9.5 (Checklist for annual review) captures Sophie's progress over the course of a year of birth-to-three services. Having these data and these displays can truly assist in showing families that change has occurred, has stalled, or even has regressed.

CONCLUSION

Monitoring progress in EI has two purposes: 1) altering and improving ongoing treatment and 2) planning for the future. Measuring performance periodically during intervention provides practitioners and caregivers with data to determine if their techniques are working and, if not, offer information about how they might be altered. Measuring performance at the end of a service delivery period provides practitioners and caregivers with information about accumulated learning and offers ideas about what might come next and planning for the future. This chapter discussed how behaviors associated with TGI can complement measures of IFSP goals for addressing these two purposes. Monitoring progress on IFSP goals will provide a picture of child change that will address broad accomplishments of significance to family needs. Examining TGI-related performance can offer a more detailed picture of change regarding the all-important areas of engagement and communication. The Checklist of Early Communication Behaviors has been recommended as a way of observing and recording engagement, communication, and cognitive change, specifically behaviors in the following areas: 1) child production of conventional preverbal communication behaviors (gaze, gestures, vocalizations), including sophistication, consistency, and independence of productions, and 2) child toy or object play with others. Details about performance in these areas can provide a more complete picture of change and contribute to decisions for altering intervention and making recommendations for the future.

Following the Triadic Gaze Intervention Journey With Children and Families

CHAPTER **10**

Triadic Gaze Intervention and Beyond

The Journey for Children and Families Continues

The first nine chapters of this book were presented in two sections: Section I (Chapters 1–3), Understanding Early Communication Development and Triadic Gaze Intervention, and Section II (Chapters 4–9), Implementing Triadic Gaze Intervention. The message underlying both parts of this book has been consistent: TGI is a strategy designed to build a foundation of preverbal behaviors that leads to successful, intentional engagement and communication for children with moderate to severe disabilities and their families. This foundation supports all kinds of early learning, but most importantly, it supports children and families in acquiring the skills needed to move forward in developing more sophisticated, conventional ways to engage and communicate. After participating in TGI, regardless of how far a child has progressed along the communication continuum, they will be poised to take the next steps in communication and language development.

The purpose of this final chapter is to begin to address the question, "What's next?" after a child and their family participate in TGI. The chapter begins with a description of the range of possibilities, with the acknowledgment that what comes next is an individual journey for each child and family, which rarely follows a linear

> TGI provides the building blocks for successful engagement and communication, from the first years of life and beyond!

path. Factors that influence how the journey may unfold, both those intrinsic to the child and those found in the extrinsic environment, are described next. These factors are not meant to be exhaustive; they are discussed with the intent to remind the practitioner of the complex variables (and interaction among these variables) that contribute to a child's lifelong journey related to communication and engagement.

Finally, this chapter concludes with stories from four families that participated in the TGI research. The decision to conclude this book with first-person accounts from families represents a conscious and deliberate shift in style and tone from previous chapters. Throughout this book, the practitioner has been guided along their own journey in learning about TGI. Important background about early communication development, detailed descriptions of the PoWRRS-Connect protocol elements, and a multitude of examples and vignettes of real-world applications of these elements have been provided. Supported with this new knowledge about TGI and the PoWRRS-Connect protocol, the practitioner now is offered the opportunity to learn from the experiences of four families who have completed their own TGI journeys, in the families' own words. Each family began their journey into communication and engagement with their children through participation in TGI and then continued to travel their unique paths with their children long after TGI ended.

This chapter is written with the strong belief and recognition that all children, regardless of which path (or paths) they take along their journey, *will* communicate and engage with their world. The hope is that this chapter and these stories will help practitioners and families recognize the value of TGI as the foundation for a variety of directions children with moderate to severe disabilities might take in learning to become successful participants when engaging with others.

HOW THE JOURNEY MAY UNFOLD

The ultimate goal of TGI is that children become intentional communicators. Until a child has learned that they can actively engage and communicate with a partner, the child will not develop advanced communication or language. There must be an intentional signal before there can be an intentional word (or symbol), phrase, or sentence. Learning that intentional signal is the very foundation provided by TGI and described in this book. But the obvious question remains: What comes next?

For all children and families, communication and engagement will continue to grow and expand well beyond their participation in TGI. What comes next, however, is unique to the child and family unit. For some, the next step may be expanded gestures or symbolic signs. For example, a child may progress from simple leaning and reaching to producing more conventional gestures, or perhaps to using manual signs or sign approximations that represent specific words and concepts. For others, next steps may include more varied or complex vocal productions, or even moving toward spoken words and sentences. For others still, next steps may involve the use of augmentative and alternative communication (AAC) systems and supports, ranging from low-tech communication boards to high-tech speech-generating devices. Note that for many children and families, next steps may include a combination of all of these communication modalities (gestures, vocalizations AAC supports/systems) employed at different times to fit the needs of a specific communication context and/or communication partner(s). The factors that may influence a child's next steps toward expanded engagement and gestural, vocal, and/or augmented communication are many. Several are discussed in the section that follows.

FACTORS THAT MAY INFLUENCE A CHILD'S JOURNEY

Both intrinsic factors (e.g., sensory/perceptual skills, gross and fine motor development, cognitive abilities, medical diagnosis) and extrinsic factors (e.g., ongoing intervention, educational experiences, familial support) may influence a child's

- Acquisition of new communication skills beyond early preverbal behaviors
- Preferred communication modality
- Ultimate success toward developing expanded communication and engagement

Of course, many of these factors are difficult to assess in children with moderate to severe disabilities, and some may never be fully known. However, it is important for the practitioner to appreciate the range and complexity of both intrinsic and extrinsic factors to better understand which ones serve as facilitators or barriers to what comes next in the child's journey toward expanded communication and engagement.

Intrinsic Factors

Factors intrinsic to the child include sensory or perceptual skills, motor skills, and cognitive abilities. Ways in which these factors might affect a child's journey and interact with one another are touched on briefly next.

Sensory and perceptual skills, such as hearing and vision, play a role in the child's preferred communication modality but often interact with motor abilities. For example, a child with a profound hearing loss likely would benefit from sign language, which is visually accessible, versus spoken language, which they cannot see or hear. A Deaf child, however, with significant cerebral palsy, may use sign language receptively with support from an interpreter but use an AAC device expressively, operating the system through a switch that maximizes some available movement. In contrast, a hearing child with cerebral palsy would be able to learn to understand speech but the oral motor challenges presented by cerebral palsy may make their own speech output unintelligible to listeners. That child could also benefit from AAC to support their expressive communication.

Oral motor skills, such as those needed for imitation and production of sounds and sound combinations, affect a child's ability to produce intelligible speech. Gross and fine motor skills affect a child's ability to develop many of the refined and intricate gestures and hand movements that compose sign language. Each of these types of potential motor skill issues, unique and intrinsic to the child, affects the child's preferred modality for expressive language.

Children diagnosed with autism compose another group with CCN; they present with unique strengths and differences that will affect their communication journey. These children often have extreme sensory or perceptual issues that affect how they receive information as well as how they express themselves and interact with those around them. For example, eye contact and physical cues such as facial expression and tone of voice are often avoided, missed, or misinterpreted by a child on the autism spectrum. Children on the autism spectrum often avoid eye contact and physical touch that are early ways of making connections with people. These various challenges will have an impact on how these children's communication journey will unfold as they move forward from the TGI foundation.

The communication path children with moderate to severe disabilities may take is also dependent on their level of cognitive functioning. For these children, knowing cognitive capacity is often a mystery because testing in this domain typically requires output that will be difficult, if not impossible, for children with moderate to severe disabilities to produce. A child's cognitive capacity will influence future learning beyond preverbal forms of communication but determining this influence will require considerable and ongoing observation and assessment.

Extrinsic Factors

Factors extrinsic to the child that influence future learning include the intervention, education, and familial support systems that surround a child after they make the transition out of birth-to-three services. These systems will vary in terms of having the resources to guide children and families through the next steps in their development of communication. Some therapeutic and educational systems will easily recognize where a child and family currently are functioning and will be able to provide the support necessary to move the child into expanded communication and engagement. Other systems may be less equipped to do so. This variability often is due to available training, financial support, and other critical resources, which often can vary based on geographical location. A number of variables clearly will influence children's next steps in communication, many of which extend beyond factors intrinsic to the child.

The stories that follow represent four different communication journeys for four different children. Each child's story highlights both intrinsic and extrinsic factors that have affected the path they have traveled. Even though we may not know which direction a child ultimately may take in learning to expand their communication and engagement, we believe that all children will find a way to communicate. These four stories exemplify this sentiment.

FOUR STORIES, FOUR COMMUNICATION JOURNEYS

The complexity of what's next following the achievement of intentional communication is as multifaceted as each child and family. The remainder of this chapter describes the unique journeys children can take, as told through the stories of four children and their families. These four children represent the variety of children seen across the three decades of TGI research. The first child was one of the four original children in the earliest study that launched the TGI program. She is the oldest of the children represented in these stories. The second child and family participated in the early parent training research. The last two children participated in research that examined practitioner training. With their TGI foundation, each of these children has moved forward to develop and expand their communication skills in a variety of ways, each unique to the child's abilities. The different stories illustrate the wide range of communication journeys and represent the role both intrinsic and extrinsic factors play in the development of communication and social engagement. Although it has been many years since these families were actively involved in TGI, each mother's description of the power and impact of the program during her time in birth-to-three services was amazing to hear and feel. The descriptions of the importance of TGI are equally strong across all four stories.

Collecting the Stories

These stories were collected via phone interviews by Dr. Gay Lloyd Pinder. The four families were chosen to represent the full 30-year span of the research program, and as such, the various research directions. The range of their children's ages (now 10–29 years) reflects the 30-year research span. When approached about their interest in having a conversation about what their child is doing now, all four mothers responded with eager pleasure to share their journeys. The conversations began by Dr. Pinder asking, "How is [child's name] doing?" and then proceeded naturally, asking for clarification and elaboration.

Each story presents a young child, almost a baby, when they started the journey through TGI with their family. It took very little encouragement to elicit the stories. Each mother spoke with positive excitement about how TGI came at a key point in their lives and what it has meant to both the child and the family over the years. No matter what the children are now doing, their mothers presented their accomplishments with pride and excitement, always going back to the TGI as the beginning of the forward movement. The stories speak for themselves and document the wide variety of paths children might follow once intentional communication has been achieved. At the end of the conversations, the stories were transcribed and then sent to the mothers for review. Each mother returned her edited version with added details or clarifications. The stories presented here are those final versions from each mother, including direct quotations (shown in italics) and Dr. Pinder's commentary.

Lauren's Story

Lauren was 13 months old when she was introduced to TGI. At that time, she had a diagnosis of hypotonia with possible cerebral palsy. She was not yet sitting independently and needed assistance to reach for and hold a toy. Lauren's older sister was 2 years old and was extremely verbal. The contrast was stark for Mother. She was struggling with helping Lauren communicate and connect with her world. She had no idea what to do with Lauren: *I was trying to lay her down under the baby gym activity center to give her stimulation, but she didn't seem to respond. She couldn't talk. She screamed when we had to ride in the car, but she couldn't tell me why, and I couldn't help her. We had to go to the medical appointments, and the appointments required long rides. It was a scary and difficult time for me. That's where we were when we met you. You gave us HOPE! Watching you work with her showed me what she could "say" with her eyes. It was like having a door open! Lauren connected with her world, and her learning took off! It was truly a miracle!*

> Watching you work with her showed me what she could "say" with her eyes. It was like having a door open! Lauren connected with her world and her learning took off!

Lauren learned triadic gaze quickly, and her signals were remarkably clear to read. Mother was like a sponge! Within 8 weeks, Lauren was making choices and requesting using eye gaze, and her mother was reading her signals like a pro! Pairing the eye gaze with gestures and vocalizations came next, and Lauren's expressive communication took off. Her mother reports: *Her ability to connect with the world started with learning how to use her eyes.* Lauren's mother truly felt that the development of Lauren's intentional communication began with triadic gaze. Lauren's journey certainly reflects the ongoing development of communication that followed. Lauren went on to learn to talk, beginning with word approximations and supplementing her early speech with some signing. Her neuromuscular issues clearly affected the intelligibility of her early speech, as did early ear infections. In time and with practice, the clarity of her speech improved, and Mother estimates that Lauren's speech is now 90% intelligible. Lauren's mother says: *She is still working on her reading skills, but her receptive and spoken vocabulary is amazing!*

Lauren is now 29 years old and "talks constantly" according to her mother. She has graduated from high school and has completed a transition program at the community college. She is living in a group home with other young adults who need assistance. Lauren works part-time as a customer service representative at a local drug store. Mother describes her as "socially driven" and states: *Her gift is her ability to interface with other people. This all started with learning to use her eyes to talk to me and me learning how to "read her eyes." It opened the door for me and for Lauren, and I want to now give back through sharing my story so other people can learn this program. This is very important to me!*

Nicole's Story

When she was born, Nicole had significant neuromuscular issues, later diagnosed as cerebral palsy; profound hearing loss that later spontaneously improved by 6 months of age, so she became aware and responsive to sound; liver failure that later spontaneously improved; and vision issues.

Nicole was 14 months old when she and her mother joined an early TGI study. At that time, Nicole did not sit up independently and was positioned in a wheelchair or in a high-chair adapted with a foam insert for stability and symmetry during the sessions. She loved to play but needed hand-over-hand assistance to manipulate toys. She moved constantly because of the cerebral palsy, and that movement made it difficult for her to stay focused visually.

Mother said that before enrolling in TGI, Nicole had no way to make choices or to communicate what she wanted. She said, *I could just give her a toy but that gave no power or opportunity to Nicole. She knew what she wanted and really needed a way to choose for herself.* She described Nicole as a child whose body and mind were so far apart! She added, *Actually, that is still true today BUT the difference now is that Nicole is able to speak for herself.*

When Nicole started the TGI at 14 months she had no way to communicate. During intervention, she learned to "quiet" her body so she could hold gaze with her eyes to choose. This was not easy for a little girl whose body was in constant motion! Mother learned how to present the choice, WAIT, and read the signal so she could honor Nicole's choice. She said: *This was new and exciting for both of us! It was a beginning.*

From that point, Nicole continued to develop her communication skills, including both sign language and speech. The family moved to Sweden for several years when Nicole was 2½. Mother explained: *In Sweden, she went to two preschools, one for kids with no disabilities and one for kids with disabilities.* There she was introduced to Blissymbols as well as Swedish sign language and spoken language, for a total of FOUR languages. According to Mother, Nicole was good at all four, and she thrived. When the family returned to the United States, Nicole was in first grade, where she learned to read with her class. She continued in general education classes and graduated from high school. As a lovely reflection of Nicole's connection to her classmates, Nicole was elected to represent her class as prom queen during her senior year.

Nicole is now 23 years old, married, and lives in an apartment with her husband. Although her body and mind continue to be far apart, Nicole uses her speech as her primary communication tool. She is speaking in full and complex sentences, but Nicole has severe athetoid cerebral palsy that affects both oral motor skills needed for articulation as well as the respiratory control needed for production of full sentences. Although her speech is not always easily intelligible to the unfamiliar listener, Nicole will work to repeat her words, and together she and the listener will come to an understanding of the meaning. Nicole is presently looking for a speech therapist with expertise in the area of cerebral palsy to work with her on her speech with focus on both oral motor precision as well as control of respiration for sound production. Nicole has begun at a community college, with a goal to find an area of interest that will enable her to find a job that will be stimulating and enable her to actively use her mind in a creative and people-focused way.

Paolo's Story

Paolo was born in 2007 and was diagnosed at birth with Down syndrome. As Paolo was growing and developing, his mom knew something was different about him when she compared his behaviors to other children with Down syndrome. She reported, *He had his own timeline for doing everything!* For example, Paolo was 4 years old before he learned to walk. Later, he was diagnosed with autism and also global apraxia. The apraxia has had a huge impact on Paolo's life because it has limited both sound production and also fine motor control.

Sign language has not been an option. Self-feeding is reportedly difficult. Dressing and undressing are also difficult. Paolo has a poor pincer grasp, and manipulative play with toys has been difficult. Paolo is unable to operate a remote with his fingers. However, in this day of tablets and screens, both of which he loves, he is learning the value of swiping.

Mom reports that the one thing Paolo really grasped was triadic eye gaze, and he has never let that go! Mother spoke with real feeling when she said, *When Paolo learned to use his eyes to communicate, his whole world opened up! He was about 15 or 16 months old when he started your program. Watching him catch on to eye gaze showed us that he really could learn. For the first time, he could tell us what he wanted. Before the triadic gaze program, Paolo would cry, and we didn't know why. Once he learned triadic gaze, when he cried, we could say, "What do you want, Paolo?" and he would immediately look at whatever he wanted and then back at us. He caught on to triadic gaze, and he has never let it go! To this day, he uses that signal. Even our friends recognize what he is saying.*

Mother described Paolo's communication: *He will make a grunting sound to get our attention. When we look, he then will look at what he wants and then back to us. If we are not in the right room, he will take us to the right room, then look at what he wants and back to us.*

> When Paolo learned to use his eyes to communicate, his whole world opened up . . . . For the first time, he could tell us what he wanted. He caught on to triadic gaze, and he has never let it go!

During this interview, we discussed where she hoped Paolo, now 13 years old, could go from here. Mother is thinking about how to expand Paolo's choices and therefore expand his communication. Music and TV are Paolo's favorite calming activities. Because of the fine motor issues, index pointing is not a strong option, so a regular communication board with little pictures has not worked. The tablet is too small for selecting items, and it does not respond to Paolo's light finger pressure. Paolo could, however, use his full hand to "point" if the pictures or board were big enough. Her plan is to use the wall in his bedroom as a communication board, beginning with four 8″ x 10″ pictures of the icons of his favorite music albums or videos. Paolo can put his hand on the picture of the song or show he wants. This was an exciting conversation of brainstorming ideas, recognizing and building on strengths, both in Paolo and in Paolo's large and active family, which includes six children (four of whom are still at home, ages 18, 13 [Paolo], 10, and 6).

For a closer look at the beginning of Paolo's journey, see Appendix C and the video of Paolo at age 11 months that accompanies the appendix.

Mateo's Story

Mateo was 18 months old when he and his mother started TGI. At that time, he was not yet sitting. His preferred position was lying on the floor watching fans and lights. He was able to roll over but had no means of mobility. He was not yet picking up toys independently but was playing hand-over-hand with others and was somewhat interested in objects, especially if he could make them spin.

Mateo's mother said she remembered one of the first TGI sessions when the clinician was working hard to encourage Mateo to pick up a toy but without success. The clinician moved him to an upright position, and the moment he was repositioned with stability provided at the hips and under his elbows, Mateo immediately reached out and tried to pick up the toy. Mother said that recognition of his positional needs was *life changing and has continued to this day.*

The next life changing moment was the actual work on eye gaze. Mother noted that *it was during the triadic gaze work that Mateo learned both the importance and also the value of making eye contact with another person.* She added that she learned how to break down communication to smaller components—how to pause and give him time to process and react. *These lessons for me made a huge difference in his learning and our communication.* Looking back, she said that the visual training was hard for Mateo because he has CVI, but no one knew that because he had not yet been diagnosed. During TGI, as Mateo learned how to use his eyes to communicate his wants, he practiced visual tracking, holding gaze on an object and then shifting gaze to make eye contact with his partner. Later, when he was finally diagnosed with CVI, he was in a position to succeed because of TGI.

There was a spark of intellect that his mother could see, but his lack of motor and vocal ability made it hard for others to appreciate. According to his mother, TGI gave Mateo a concrete way to make his presence and his thoughts known, and for that she will be forever grateful! Mother said, *Mateo is now 10 years old, and he still uses triadic gaze to communicate with me today! He will get my attention by making eye contact. He learned that with you all!* She indicated that Mateo does not use speech at all, but rather he uses triadic gaze with a variety of gestures and a few signs. He slaps his chest to say "I" or Mateo. His signs include BATH, MUSIC, MORE, and MILK. Mother said Mateo does not nod or shake his head reliably to say yes or no. Instead, he smiles or does a dance to say "yes." For "no," he will push an item away or simply ignore you. When he wants something, Mateo, who is now ambulatory with steadily improving balance, will either bring you to the item or bring the item to you. For example, if he wants to go out, Mateo will bring Mother's coat or backpack to her. If he is hungry, he will bring Mother to the fridge. Mother is working with Mateo to teach him to point for himself.

Mother added, *I learned two huge things working with the TGI team: 1) The TGI program taught me how to play with him, and 2) TGI taught me how to "read" him.* She said, *That was the beginning of our real communication with Mateo. We learned how to interact with him, and we learned how to connect with him.* Progress has continued one small step at a time! For many years, Mother reported trying unsuccessfully to interest Mateo in reading books. *Just recently, for the very first time, Mateo brought a favorite book to me to read to him! That was a gift to me!*

The family recently moved, and Mateo is now in a new school system with a new team, in which his mother has increasing confidence. Having this confidence in Mateo's team is new and exciting for her. Because of COVID-19, Mateo is now at home doing online school with his teacher; the home activities are supervised by his mother. Mother is very impressed by both the creativity and proactive approach of Mateo's teacher, the SLP, and the vision specialist. Her confidence in the new team has the potential to enhance Mateo's program and progress in a positive way.

The SLP first got a tablet for Mateo and has now introduced a communication app with voice output. Mateo presses a picture or symbol, and the tablet speaks the word. If he presses several pictures or symbols to make a sentence, the communication app will say the sentence (e.g., "I want _____"). The SLP is making it worth Mateo's effort by using his favorite music and videos. Mother said this is giving him a sense of what it can do for him. Mother is always present during the sessions and is thus able to interpret some of Mateo's subtle communication cues. For example, one day as they were playing with the tablet using his communication app, Mateo made a negative sound, seeming to say "no." When the SLP stopped the video, Mother clarified Mateo's negative "no" sound, saying, *He didn't mean "Turn it off." He meant "No, don't stop!" In other words, "leave it on."* Mateo is learning to expand his expressive communication skills through operating a device with voice output to potentially communicate with people outside his immediate family.

CONCLUSION

This chapter ends with stories from four mothers of children with moderate to severe disabilities who have lived the early support journey. The stories capture the wide range of abilities and disabilities that characterize children with CCN. Yet, despite the differences among children, all of the stories start out the same. The stories begin with the mothers reflecting on the early frustration of not being able to connect with their children. The children were stuck, and the families were stuck in not knowing how to engage and communicate with each other. TGI served as a strategy to offer a direct and pragmatic way to focus on this challenge within the families' daily routines. The stories provide testaments about the power of TGI for building foundational behaviors that led to intentional preverbal behaviors and later to expanded communication behaviors of various forms. Simply put, both families and children learned the power of gaze, gestures, and vocalization for expressing wants and needs. They also learned the power of these behaviors for providing the building blocks for all kinds of engagement and developing communication. The intensity of these mothers' stories gives credence to the powerful and lasting importance of TGI to both the children and their families.

The four stories also serve as an exemplary ending for this book. The stories bring the themes of this book full circle and authenticate the following nine key take-home messages:

1. Communication begins before words. Preverbal behaviors (gaze, gestures, vocalizations) compose the conventional forms of these early communication signals that help children and families engage with one another.

2. Intentional communication emerges along a continuum, where children learn to link focus on people and objects to demonstrate their wants and needs. The developmental continuum moves from single, to dual, to triadic focus—the latter of which has marked intentionality. As these gaze behaviors develop, gestures and vocalizations add to increased sophistication, clarity, and control.

3. Intentional preverbal communication is the foundation for intentional symbolic forms of communication: signs, spoken words, and augmentative and alternative forms.

4. Early in life, families are the most important communication partners for their children.

5. A supportive caregiver–practitioner partnership builds caregiver confidence and sets the stage for the success of TGI.

6. TGI is a strategy to help families understand how to best build the foundational skills for engagement and communication as well as future learning.

7. TGI is flexible in its implementation, adapting to different child characteristics, family beliefs, resources, and daily routines.

8. The PoWRRS-Connect protocol used to implement TGI can be delivered anytime, anywhere, and by anyone. The six elements of PoWRRS-Connect: **provide opportunity**, **wait**, **recognize** the child's communication attempt, **respond** to that attempt, when appropriate **shape** the attempt to a more sophisticated form, and **connect** can and should become second nature to families. Although deliberate, the protocol is a natural and comfortable way to interact.

9. Anywhere a child lands on the continuum in learning intentional communication will provide them with the foundation to move to the next step in communication, whatever direction that may be.

As this book ends, we reflect on the importance of engagement and communication in our lives as well as the significance of providing children with the support they need to develop skills in these areas. For children with disabilities and CCN, disruption in engagement and early communication can be a significant hindrance during the first years of life. The resulting loss in connections with others can jeopardize relationships and future learning. Children struggle and families struggle; however, we believe these children and their families can learn to read each other and connect. We presume that with dedicated guidance children and their families can be successful communicators with one another. As we face the current pandemic crisis, we pause to consider how challenges in engagement and communication might be weighing even more heavily on these families. As professionals who participate in early intervention, we are obligated to find ways to help. Given our expertise, we are obligated to share our knowledge with families and offer appropriate guidance. We offer the information in this book about TGI as our way to assist children and their families as they engage and communicate with one another.

Triadic Gaze Intervention Research Program and Supporting Evidence

Over nearly three decades, a series of studies conducted at the University of Washington, Department of Speech and Hearing Sciences, has investigated the benefits of Triadic Gaze Intervention (TGI) with children with moderate to severe disabilities and complex communication needs. This body of evidence is reviewed from the earliest feasibility studies to the most recent research investigating implementation of the protocol in practice.

FEASIBILITY STUDIES

The first research was a series of time series studies to explore an early form of treatment designed to teach potentially communicative behaviors of gaze, gestures, and vocalizations. In the first study, Pinder and colleagues (1993) conducted a case study to explore the feasibility of administering a treatment that emphasized providing children with opportunities to communicate and shaping their behaviors toward conventional gaze, gestural, and vocal behaviors, which led to triadic gaze. This study examined the child's learning in different contexts (request and choice). The 20-month-old child, who had severe physical impairments with a diagnosis of cerebral palsy, was enrolled in treatment conducted by a speech-language pathologist (SLP) in a clinic setting for approximately 5 months. The within (ABA) and between (multiple baseline across request and choice context) series design demonstrated that the child responded well to the treatment and learned to produce a variety of communicative behaviors (including dual and triadic focus) in play activities that offered opportunities for both requesting and choosing. Triadic gaze appeared to be more successfully produced in the request context.

For more information, see

- Pinder, G. L., Olswang, L., & Coggins, K. (1993). The development of communicative intent in a physically disabled child. *Infant-Toddler Intervention, 3,* 1–17.

The next research (Pinder & Olswang, 1995) replicated the case study by examining the treatment with four different children ages 11.5–13.5 months diagnosed with cerebral palsy. The children's motor impairments were characterized as moderate to severe. In this study, the teaching context and length of treatment were investigated more thoroughly in a within (ABA) and between (multiple baseline across participants) series single-subject design with multiple measures. As with the first case study, treatment was administered by a single SLP in a clinic setting. All of the children learned to produce more conventional communicative behaviors, although individual differences in success with particular behaviors were noted, along with length of time to show change. The research was instrumental in showing that opportunities for requesting during play were most successful in eliciting communicative behaviors. In addition to examining communicative behaviors as an outcome measure, play with toys was also investigated through quantitative and qualitative measures. Results demonstrated that the treatment appeared to encourage more and longer periods of toy exploration and manipulation. They showed more variety and sophistication in their object play and more involvement with the adult. The children increased their visual regard for objects, examining toys from a variety of angles. They explored objects through a variety of manipulations, including rubbing, squeezing, and banging toys. They gradually seemed to learn about object parts and their locative and functional relations. Most significantly, the children increased their effort to engage the adult in object play routines. They appeared to learn that adults could be a means to ends. The observed changes in object play paralleled the development of communication behaviors.

For more information, see

- Pinder, G. L., & Olswang, L. (1995). Development of communicative intent in young children with cerebral palsy: A treatment efficacy study. *Infant-Toddler Intervention, 5,* 51–69.

- Olswang, L., & Pinder, G. L. (1995). Preverbal functional communication and the role of object play in children with cerebral palsy. *Infant-Toddler Intervention, 5,* 277–300.

The preliminary success of TGI led us to want to work more closely with caregivers. In the next research project, three caregivers of children (age 14–21 months) diagnosed with cerebral palsy and severe motor impairments participated in the intervention. We taught caregivers to administer the treatment protocol over a 3-week period. The treatment protocol in this study had evolved to include specific elements, consisting of providing communication opportunities, waiting for a child response, acknowledging the child's attempt, and trying to shape a clearer signal. An SLP instructed the caregivers in the administration of the protocol, using modeling with practice and feedback. We measured caregiver learning and child communication. Caregivers successfully learned to produce the treatment elements; however, the degree of success varied across caregivers and across individual elements. Caregivers easily learned how to provide opportunities and wait for a child response. They had more difficulty acknowledging and shaping their children's communicative attempts. All children showed improved communication (dual and triadic focus) with their caregivers during the 3-week period and afterward. This study was influential in understanding that different aspects of the protocol were harder to learn than others for caregivers.

For more information, see

- Olswang, L., Pinder, G. L., & Hanson, R. (2006). Communication in young children with motor impairments: Teaching caregivers to teach. *Seminars in Speech and Language, 27,* 199–214.

CASE-CONTROLLED STUDY

Between 2006 and 2012, our research was part of a program project funded through the National Institutes of Health, Child Health and Human Development, in collaboration with colleagues at the University of Kansas who were exploring nonverbal communication behaviors in separate populations (adults with severe disabilities and preschool children with complex communication needs). In our collaboration, we continued examining the efficacy of TGI with very young children with moderate to severe disabilities and complex communication needs using a randomized controlled study. This project resulted in the exploration of several aspects of TGI. First, we more fully defined gaze, gestural, and vocal behaviors and described them as a continuum of emerging pre-intentional to intentional communication prior to first words and symbols. Second, we more fully defined the treatment protocol used to implement TGI so that reliability in administration by different SLPs could be documented along with the efficacy of the treatment. PoWRRS-Connect became the acronym for the six essential elements of the protocol: provide opportunity, wait, recognize the child's behavior, respond, shape, and connect. Third, we explored the validity of assessment procedures as a way to predict the benefits of TGI.

The research documenting the emergence of nonverbal communication behaviors resulted in the development of the Communication Complexity Scale (CCS) (Brady et al., 2012). The CCS is a tool for assessing nonverbal communication behaviors leading to first words across different populations with severe disabilities (infants, preschoolers, and adults who are nonverbal). We documented the validity of this tool, which serves as the child behavior continuum that guides treatment for TGI. As this book is being written, research addressing the standardization of this assessment instrument is continuing.

For more information, see

- Brady, N., Fleming, K., Thiemann-Bourke, K., Olswang, L., Dowden, P., & Saunders, M. (2012). Development of the Communication Complexity Scale. *American Journal of Speech-Language Pathology, 21,* 16–28.

The primary focus of the randomized controlled study examined TGI versus standard care or treatment in 18 children between 10 and 24 months with moderate to severe disabilities and complex communication needs. Children in the TGI group received services via three different SLPs implementing the PoWRRS-Connect protocol in the natural environment. Children in the standard care group received services through birth-to-three centers in either center or natural environments. Results documented that children who received TGI treatment (experimental group) demonstrated greater peak performance in triadic gaze behaviors than children who received early standard care treatment (control group). However, individual differences in child change were also documented.

For more information, see

- Olswang, L. B., Dowden, P., Feuerstein, J., Greenslade, K., Pinder, G. L., & Fleming, K. (2014). Triadic gaze intervention for young children with physical disabilities. *Journal of Speech-Language, and Hearing Research, 57,* 1740–1753.

Another important outcome of this program project was the examination of the heterogeneity of learning triadic gaze through PoWRRS-Connect. The progress of six children in the research was examined in relationship to dynamic assessment procedures (abbreviated form of PoWRRS-Connect) conducted prior to treatment. This research demonstrated the validity of dynamic assessment for predicting change in the children's learning triadic gaze through PoWRRS-Connect. Furthermore, this research explored whether the assessment procedures could provide guidance regarding which preverbal behaviors (dual focus or triadic focus) should be targeted in treatment.

For more information, see

- Olswang, L., Feuerstein, J., Pinder, G. L., & Dowden, P. (2013). Validating dynamic assessment of triadic gaze for young children with severe disabilities. *American Journal of Speech-Language Pathology, 22,* 449–462.

IMPLEMENTATION STUDIES

As we considered further exploring TGI, particularly in light of individual differences in child outcomes, we decided to do so in the context of clinical practice. This implementation research, employing both quantitative and qualitative methodology, was funded by the University of Washington, Institute of Translational Health Sciences, with a particular emphasis on the practitioner's role in administering TGI. A significant aspect of this research was manualizing the TGI strategy, including the following information: 1) providing background information on early communication and a rationale for prioritizing engagement and communication in services to families, and 2) describing the six elements of the PoWRRS-Connect protocol and instructing practitioners on its implementation. The research explored practitioner fidelity in delivering the PoWRRS-Connect protocol and their views on adopting TGI in their clinical routines. The research included seven early intervention clinicians from multiple disciplines (occupational therapist, physical therapist, SLP). The first study demonstrated practitioners' abilities to accurately administer the six elements of the PoWRRS-Connect protocol. It also demonstrated diversity in quality of administration, with corresponding impact on child performance. The second study revealed strengths and weaknesses to incorporating TGI into early intervention practice. Strengths included the transdisciplinary approach of TGI, the focus and structure of TGI, and the ease of incorporating the PoWRRS-Connect protocol into typical treatment routines. The weaknesses included challenges in using data collection forms. Another important outcome of this research was the consensus among clinicians that we should disseminate the TGI strategy more broadly with EI professionals and caregivers. This research was particularly informative for shaping the content of this book.

For more information, see

- Feuerstein, J., Olswang, L., Greenslade, K., Pinder, G. L., Dowden, P., & Madden, J. (2017). Moving triadic gaze intervention into practice: Measuring clinician attitude and implementation fidelity. *Journal of Speech, Language, and Hearing Research, 60*(5), 1285–1298.

- Feuerstein, J., Olswang, L., Greenslade, K., Dowden, P., Pinder, G. L., & Madden, J. (2018). Implementation research: Embracing practitioners' views. *Journal of Speech, Language, and Hearing Research, 61,* 645–657.

The final piece of evidence involved a training study. This research investigated teaching aspects of PoWRRS-Connect to EI speech-language pathologists using an online training platform, specifically recognizing preverbal communication behaviors. Using a randomized controlled trial, we compared three online conditions: practice with implicit problem solving, practice with explicit problem solving, or no practice. We examined knowledge about early communication, skill at recognizing preverbal behaviors, time taken to complete the training, and perceptions of the training experience. The study demonstrated the no-practice control condition took significantly less time to complete during the training, achieved the same positive outcomes on the knowledge and skill assessments, and was rated as appealing as the other conditions. These results provided important information about efficiency, appeal, and effectiveness of specific online training strategies for TGI and PoWRRS-Connect.

For more information, see

- Feuerstein, J., & Olswang, L. (2020). A randomized controlled trial investigating online training for prelinguistic communication. *Journal of Speech, Language, and Hearing Research, 63,* 827–833.

Checklist of Early Communication Behaviors

Note: The Checklist is also available for download at the Brookes Download Hub along with other online resources for this book.

Checklist of Early Communication Behaviors

Name:

Foundational Behaviors for Triadic Gaze			Source of Information		Notes
			Caregiver Reported	Practitioner Observed	Activity or Routine, Toys or Objects, People Present, Prompts Used
Gaze	Single Focus	Looks and sustains gaze to a **person***			
		Looks and sustains gaze to an **object***			
		Follows a moving **object***			
	Dual Focus	Looks back and forth between **two objects***			
		Looks from **object to person OR person to object***			
	Triadic Focus	Looks **back and forth** between object **AND** person*			
Vocalizations		Produces **early sounds** (fusses, squeals)			
		Produces **consonants, vowels,** and **consonant– vowel combinations**			
		Produces **word approximations**			
Gestures		**Leans/reaches** for object **OR** person*			
		Shows, points, gives			
		Uses **gestures** meaningfully (waves hi/bye, covers eyes for Peekaboo)			

*NOTE: Be sure to note if the child also uses vocalizations and/or gestures when looking.

Building Preverbal Communication & Engagement: Triadic Gaze Intervention for Young Children With Disabilities and Their Families
by Lesley B. Olswang, Julie L. Feuerstein, and Gay Lloyd Pinder. Copyright © 2022 by Paul H. Brookes Publishing Co., Inc. All rights reserved.

APPENDIX C

Video Exemplars of PoWRRS-Connect

The three video exemplars in this appendix illustrate the six elements of PoWRRS-Connect, when put together. When reviewing these videos, note both child and adult behaviors. (Elements of PoWRRS-Connect shown in bold type in this appendix are defined in the glossary. Video descriptions include approximate time indications when certain behaviors are demonstrated within each video clip.) In all three of these videos, the adult is a speech-language pathologist (SLP). These video segments have been used to model PoWRRS-Connect to families and practitioners.

VIDEO 1: MARLEY

The first treatment video shows a 19-month-old female, Marley, with the following characteristics:

- *Diagnosis:* Unknown

- *Hearing:* Corrected with aids

- *Muscle tone:* Hypotonic

- *Gross motor:* Independent sitting—Treatment was primarily conducted in a highchair.

- *Other:* Various orthopedic needs

- *Communicative signals and motor behaviors:* Reaching, clapping, limited vocalizations

- *Interests:* Equal interest in objects and adults

In this video, you will see the SLP offer four opportunities, several of which are discussed in detail next:

a. 0:06: Choice (yogurt snack, book)

b. 1:05: Request (more book)

c. 2:04: Choice (yogurt snack, book)

d. 3:05: Request (more book)

The first portion of the video demonstrates using PoWRRS-Connect during snack and toy play. Mom informed the SLP that Marley might want a snack, so the SLP started the session with a **choice opportunity** (0:06) between a snack item and a book.

First, the SLP presents both items; Marley looks at each item and back up at the SLP.

- The SLP **recognizes** and acknowledges Marley's looking.

- Then, the SLP verbally prompts Marley to look at the one she wants, saying, "Good finding my eyes; now look at your choice."

- The SLP **waits**, and after approximately 3 seconds Marley looks at the book, indicating her choice.

- Because this session occurred early in Marley's treatment, the SLP was encouraging dual focus—looking between the object and an adult.

- Notice how the SLP **shapes**, telling Marley to use her eyes and reinforcing her effort by giving her the book and telling her, "You used your eyes to say, I want that book!"

- Notice, too, how the **choice opportunity** ends with the SLP reading with the child. This reinforces the child's communication gaze behavior.

Marley's apparent interest in the book leads the SLP to set up a **request opportunity** for "more" (1:05). Notice how naturally the request flows from the previous choice opportunity and connecting.

Next, the SLP presents the book and asks, "Do you want more book?"

- Marley looks at the book and claps her hands to midline.

- The SLP **waits** (almost 10 seconds!) before using a verbal prompt ("Marley!") to get the child to look back at her.

- Once Marley looks at the SLP, she asks, "Do you want more?"

- She also nicely **responds** and reinforces gaze directly: "Good looking. Thank you for telling me 'more' with your eyes!"

Notice again the **connection**/playing at the end with the book reading.

Finally, at the end of the segment, the SLP presents the book in a **request opportunity** (3:05). In response, Marley produces a triadic gaze as her final behavior. She seems to have the idea of using her eyes to communicate ("You found my eyes. Good looking back at the book to tell me more. Yea, your eyes did that, Marley. I was watching!") and the adult is **recognizing** this behavior, **responding** to it as an intentional communication, and reinforcing it with **connecting**—illustrating the full PoWRRS-Connect.

You might wonder if Marley's clapping is an attempt to sign more. She often claps her hands together when the SLP says "more," but she is not consistent in doing so. She might have a sense that this is a signal of excitement and even participation, but there is no indication that the behavior is used to communicate intentionally.

VIDEO 2: PAOLO

The second treatment video shows an 11-month-old male, Paolo, with the following characteristics:

- *Diagnosis:* Down syndrome

- *Muscle tone:* Hypotonic

- *Gross motor:* Independent sitting—Treatment was conducted in a highchair or on the floor.

- *Other:* Feeding problems (at the beginning of treatment)

- *Communicative signals and motor behaviors:* Reaching, holding toys, banging toys, vocalizing

- *Interests:* Primarily interested in looking at and playing with people; limited attention to objects

In this video, you will see the SLP offer five opportunities, several of which are discussed in detail next:

a. 0:10: Request (more ball)

b. 0:38: Choice (ball, truck)

c. 1:45: Choice (truck, ball)

d. 2:15: Choice (puppy, squishy ball)

e. 3:30: Request (more squishy ball)

This segment starts with Paolo playing with a "ball" that he can hold and shake. The bell inside the ball helps to get and maintain his attention. As you see, Paolo seems to like the toy. The SLP engages him in play and uses her turn to move the ball out of his reach and creates a **request opportunity** (0:10).

- The SLP holds the ball to the side, directly asking, "Shall we do more?"

- The SLP **waits** for Paolo to look at the ball, but he focuses on her, vocalizes, and sustains his gaze to her only. This behavior might be a request for more, but the SLP wants to **shape** a more sophisticated behavior: looking between the ball and her (dual focus).

- The SLP shakes the ball to get his attention back to the object, but without luck.

- The SLP moves the ball to the other side and provides verbal prompts ("You can use your eyes to tell me! Look back at the ball for more") but Paolo's gaze remains stuck on her. Although Paolo might glance at the ball, he never convincingly looks back at it. Paolo continues to vocalize and reaches toward the adult, which she **recognizes** and acknowledges.

The SLP's next move is a good one; she uses his distraction as an opportunity to bring him back to toy play. She introduces a new toy, the truck, in a **choice opportunity** (0:38).

- *Notice:* The SLP gets him to look at each toy. First, she shakes and taps the ball on the table, while labeling it. Then, she shakes the truck and labels it, holding both up and saying, "Which?" Paolo looks at the truck and back up at her.

- She uses a verbal prompt to get him to look back at the truck ("Which?").

- She clearly reinforces his using his eyes to make a choice, stating: "Your eyes told me truck!"); this was a beautifully **shaped** triadic gaze.

- This is followed by a nice play moment with the truck, demonstrating the various parts (wheels) and possible actions (rolling, spinning), all while following his lead.

The SLP again uses the natural toy play, when the truck gets dropped on the side of the highchair, to introduce another **choice opportunity** (1:45).

- She again presents the truck and the ball because he had shown interest in both toys earlier.

- *Note:* She holds up each toy at eye level, shaking and labeling each.

Paolo's lack of interest leads her to present a new toy, the puppy dog, which she then pairs with a squishy ball (a toy he had shown interest in during a previous session) in another **choice opportunity** (2:15).

- *Notice here:* He looks at both objects, then goes back to the squishy ball and looks up at the SLP.

- The SLP uses this as a chance to try to **shape** a full triadic gaze. She tells him to "look back at the ball" and moves the ball up toward her face.

- When Paolo looks back at the puppy, she legitimately acknowledges that maybe he changed his mind. This is a good example of showing him that he is not communicating clearly.

- The SLP offers the choice again but switches the toys' positions to make sure she has his attention and is giving him a clear choice.

- She **recognizes** and acknowledges his looking at the ball and then her.

- Then, she uses verbal and visual prompts to get him to look at the ball again, thus ending by reinforcing a **shaped** triadic gaze.

- Play with the squishy ball follows.

Again, the ball dropping off the tray provides a natural opportunity to reintroduce it using a **request opportunity** (3:30).

- This opportunity ends with Paolo producing a nice triadic gaze.

VIDEO 3: BENJAMIN

The third treatment video shows a male, Benjamin, around 18–20 months of age, with the following characteristics:

- *Diagnosis:* Cerebral palsy (athetoid)

- *Muscle tone:* Hypotonic to fluctuating

- *Gross motor:* No independent sitting; no rolling

- Treatment with SLP alone was conducted in a highchair adapted with a foam insert to provide additional hip and pelvic stability.

- Co-treatment with SLP and occupational therapist (OT) was conducted in a variety of positions with movement.

- *Other:* Feeding difficulties; visual acuity improved with glasses

- *Communicative signals and motor behaviors:* Eye movement (e.g., eye contact, visual tracking); vocalization with effort and increased tone; extreme difficulty with coordinated reach; unable to maintain grasp on toys or to point

- *Interests:* Interested in both objects and adults

History: At the beginning of treatment, Mom and the SLP were hoping to increase Benjamin's gaze and reaching as a communication signal. It was quickly apparent that his physical disabilities prevented him from reaching successfully. When he became excited or attempted to reach, his muscle tone increased, and his arm would pull back. His eyes were the most dependable part of Benjamin's body. For that reason, the SLP and Mom shifted their focus to teaching Benjamin to use his eyes for communication purposes.

During this play interaction, the objective was to encourage behaviors that make up triadic gaze: looking at objects, looking at the adult, and linking the two by scanning between object and adult. Benjamin's physical disabilities required that he have considerable support so he could fully participate. This video illustrates co-treatment, meaning two practitioners are working collaboratively with the child: The one in front (an SLP) is communicating and playing with the child, and the one behind (an OT) is physically supporting him. The therapy ball that Benjamin is positioned on is used to support his trunk and maximize his opportunities for engagement during play.

During this video segment, you will see the SLP use verbal, visual, tactile, and auditory prompts to encourage Benjamin to look down to locate each block, then visually track the block as it moves up the ball (**shaping**). She presents each opportunity for Benjamin to use his eyes in this way by saying, "Should we get another one?" These become opportunities for Benjamin to begin to learn requesting.

Note the following during these opportunities (0:32, 1:06, 1:44):

- The SLP is positioned at midline, at Benjamin's eye level, and close to his face.

- The SLP carefully paces the movement of the block, so Benjamin is able to maintain gaze and watch the block all the way up the ball.

- The SLP comments or asks a question (**requesting opportunities**), then **waits** to allow Benjamin time to gather himself to respond, either taking a breath to vocalize or controlling his body to smile. She also **recognizes** and **responds** to his attempts to participate and communicate.

Each block becomes a practice moment, including looking at the object, tracking the object, looking at the SLP, and playing with the blocks.

- Stacking is a typical and fun way for exploring objects, but Benjamin's cerebral palsy presented obstacles to having these early play experiences. The block play was new and exciting for him and became possible in the co-treatment session.

- The OT provided the foundation in the postural control through his trunk, while the SLP worked with his shoulders and arms, allowing Benjamin to respond to the play situation.

- As you watch the video, note how Benjamin "reaches," and the SLP keeps his arm forward, preventing the elbow from bending and pulling back.

- Then, the OT supports at the back of the shoulder, allowing the SLP to guide his arm/hand to participate in stacking the block.

- The repetition helps the child in two ways: 1) gaining physical strength so that at the end he is able to take weight on his arms and hold his head up to look at his stack of blocks, and 2) learning to engage with the SLP and use his eyes and vocalizations to communicate his desire to keep playing. The latter reflects coordinated joint attention and the component behaviors of triadic gaze, which reinforce cognitive development of means/ends relationships.

- At the conclusion of the video, watch how Benjamin looks down to the blocks spontaneously after knocking the tower over (4:47)! The OT **recognizes** and **responds**, reinforcing this gaze behavior by saying, "Nice looking!"

Although this video illustrates two practitioners working with the child, caregivers certainly can play either role with guidance from a professional.

Handouts for Families

1. Early Communication in Typical Development

2. PoWRRS-Connect: How to Help Your Child Engage and Communicate

Early Communication in Typical Development

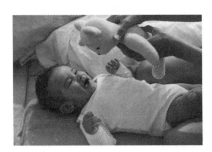

A lot of communication can happen before children produce their first words or signs. Early conventional signals include *gaze* (looking/staring), *gestures* (leaning, reaching), and *vocalizations* (simple sounds). The Early Communication chart in the next section explains more about these conventional signals of early communication. Recognizing and responding to these signals encourages children to use them again and again. Gradually their signals become clearer and more purposeful.

How do early conventional signals of engagement and communication develop?

In the first months, babies typically show an interest in objects and adults. They actively look at each one separately. Usually if a child is looking at an object, you look at the object, too. You might even name the object ("That's juice!") or ask a question about the object ("Do you want the juice?").

The child gradually begins to link the adult and object by looking first at one, then at the other. By looking back and forth between the adult and object, the child can clearly communicate a message. Sometimes that message may be a request, such as "I want the blocks," while looking at the blocks, back to you, and then back to the blocks. Other times the baby may be making a comment, such as "Look, doggy doggy!" as observed by their expression of excitedly looking between you and the family dog. Sometimes, if you give a child a choice by holding up two items, such as juice and cracker, a child can pick the one they want by looking.

Sometimes young children will make sounds or gestures as they look; maybe something that sounds like *da* for "that," or *mu* for "more," while leaning or even reaching. These behaviors can help make the message even clearer.

As children get better at looking, making sounds, and gesturing, we have an easier time understanding their signals. We seem to have a better idea of what the baby is trying to tell us.

Your child may have trouble producing early signals, which may mean you have a hard time knowing what your child wants.

Sometimes signals may appear but then disappear. Sometimes your child may cry or fuss, which is a signal, but these signals can be frustrating because they may be difficult to interpret. Maybe there are better signals. Learning conventional signals, such as those listed in the chart below, and how to help encourage them will be a big part of early intervention.

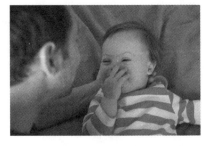

Early Communication

Gaze	Single Focus	Looks and sustains gaze to a **person**
		Looks and sustains gaze to an **object**
		Follows a moving **object**
	Dual Focus	Looks back and forth between **two objects**
		Looks from **object to person OR person to object**
	Triadic Focus	Looks **back and forth** between object **AND** person
Vocalizations		Produces **early sounds** (fusses, squeals, coos)
		Produces **consonants, vowels**, and **consonant–vowel combinations of various types** (*bu bu bu, bubu, mubu, da, dada*)
		Produces **word approximations** (*mo* for "more," *bubu* for "bye bye")
Gestures		**Leans/reaches** for object **OR** person
		Shows, points, gives
		Uses **gestures** meaningfully (waves hi/bye, covers eyes for Peekaboo)

Remember . . .

Each type of behavior (gaze, gesture, and vocalization) emerges over time, but they also come together!

Children are different in how they communicate!

Some children may produce behaviors clearly—others may not.
Some children may produce behaviors quickly—others more slowly.

TRIADIC GAZE INTERVENTION

PoWRRS-Connect

HOW TO HELP YOUR CHILD ENGAGE
AND COMMUNICATE

1. PROVIDE AN OPPORTUNITY

Show your child something interesting.
  (A favorite toy or snack)
Start a favorite game.
  (Peekaboo with a scarf)
Pause and ask:
  Which one do you want? (two toy or snack options)
  Do you want more? (hold up the scarf)

2. WAIT AND WATCH

Give your child time to respond.
  Try counting to five in your head!
Watch what your child does:
  What do they look at (gaze)?
  What do they lean or reach toward (gesture)?
  What sounds do they make (vocalization)?

3. RECOGNIZE THEIR SIGNALS

Gaze: Looking at objects and/or people
Gestures: Leaning, tilting, reaching
Vocalizations: Making sounds (maybe even words!)

4. RESPOND

Say what your child is doing:
  You're looking at juice; I bet you want it!
  You're leaning toward the doggy!
  You want the doggy!

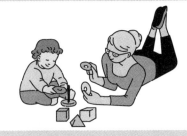

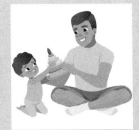

5. SHAPE

Try to get a clearer signal.
Say and show what to do:
  Say: "You looked at juice; now look back at me!"
  Show: by moving the juice cup (or bottle) up to your eyes

CONNECT DURING EVERYDAY MOMENTS

Practice during routines such as play, snack, bath, or mealtime. . .
But most importantly, have fun with your child!

Activity	What you do: PROVIDE AN OPPORTUNITY and WAIT		What your CHILD might do (signals)	How you might RESPOND/SHAPE
	Offer a request or choice	Wait		
Musical toys • You ring a bell, shake a rattle, or hit a drum. • Hold your child's hand so they can play along. • Try to get your child to look at the toy—the sound of the toy can help!	**Request for more:** **Say:** "Look at the bell," "Ring ring," or "Look at the rattle," "Shake shake." **Ask:** "Do you want me to ring it again?" or "Do you want me to shake it again?" Hold the toy up so it is easy to see but just out of reach.	Wait and watch	Your child *looks* away or puts their head down. This signal is hard to read. You might wonder, is your child interested? Or maybe you wonder if your child knows how to use eye gaze to signal.	You might try again to see if you can get your child to look at the toy. Ring the bell, and **say,** "Listen, ring, ring; look at the bell." You might help your child touch the toy and help you play with it. Be patient and try again. If there is any interest—play with the toy again. Describe your child's looking. Doing this slowly and repeatedly is just fine! Maybe your child wants another toy. Your child might fuss or turn away. Then, try a different toy. Toys that make sounds can help a child to look. Toys that provide lights are good too for helping your child attend.
Stacking blocks • You are helping your child stack blocks (hand over hand). • You may help your child knock them over.	**Request for more:** After you knock the blocks over: **Ask:** "Do you want more blocks?" Hold one block up when your child can see it. Maybe you will need to stack one and then hold up another.	Wait and watch	Your child *looks* at the blocks and even seems to *lean* toward them. Your child might even seem excited. This is a clear signal!	You could **say,** "You are looking at the blocks. You're trying to get them. You're telling me you want more blocks." Wait a little bit, then bring the block close to your eyes, and see if your child looks at you, too. Make sure you end with stacking the blocks.

Activity	What you do: PROVIDE AN OPPORTUNITY and WAIT		What your CHILD might do (signals)	How you might RESPOND/SHAPE
	Offer a request or choice	Wait		
Snack time with cereal and juice • You are giving your child a snack.	**Choice:** **Say:** "Look, your favorites, cereal and juice." **Ask:** "Which one do you want?" Hold up both, one in each hand, so your child can easily see them, but just out of reach. You can describe each one if you want. Make sure your child sees each one. You might have to help get their attention.	Wait and watch	Your child only looks at one. You want to make sure your child has seen both. Slowly move each one. Finally, your child looks at the juice and makes a sound. This is a clear signal!	Your waiting allowed your child to make a choice. Vocalizing helps to make the signal clear. **Say,** "You're looking at the juice; you must want it." Give your child a sip of juice. Try this whole series again. After your child looks at one of the items, move it toward your face to see if they might look at you, too. If looking happens, make sure you describe it. Say, "You're looking at the juice and at me. You're telling me you want the juice."
Scarf Peekaboo • You put a scarf over your baby's head and say, "Where's baby?" then pull the scarf off and say "Peekaboo!" • Repeat a couple of times.	**Request:** **Say:** "That was fun." Hold the scarf up so your child can see it, but out of reach. **Ask:** "Do you want more Peekaboo?" After a couple of Peekaboo games, add a new toy for a choice. **Choice:** Hold up the scarf in one hand and a familiar toy (e.g., favorite rattle with lion) in the other hand. Make sure your child can see both but cannot grab them. **Ask:** "Do you want to play Peekaboo again, or play with the lion rattle?"	Wait and watch	**Request:** Your child looks at the scarf and tries to reach. This is a clear signal. Use it to build another opportunity. **Choice:** Your child looks at the scarf and then looks at the new toy. Your child settles on the new toy, reaching and vocalizing.	You could say, "You're looking and reaching for the scarf. You want to play again." Repeat the Peekaboo game. Maybe try to get your child to look at you, too. You could say, "Oh, now you want to play with your lion rattle. Can you look at Mommy/Daddy, too?" You hold the rattle close to your eyes, and as your child follows it, you comment, "Yes, you're looking at your favorite rattle and at Mommy/Daddy. Here you go!" Give the rattle to your child. It is fun to mix choice and request!

These are just examples. What exactly you say and how your baby responds will be different. The main idea is to play with your child, pause/stop the activity, and ask if your child would like more or ask which activity your child would like and wait for them to respond. Watch their eyes to see if you can encourage looking between you and the desired object. Then, respond to your child by either starting the activity back up if they want more, or changing an activity if the child indicate they are done.

Glossary

actual level of performance Level of skill or behavior at which the child is currently functioning without adult assistance. *See also* potential level of performance.

authentic routines Routines that refer to practices and activities that naturally occur in families' daily lives. *See also* routines-based intervention (RBI).

caregivers Individuals responsible for the primary care of children: biological, adopted, or foster. These can include parents, grandparents, other relatives, babysitters/nannies, or teachers.

choice opportunity An opportunity to communicate where two items (e.g., objects/toys, food items) are offered to a child and the child is expected to choose one over the other. *See also* PoWRRS-Connect; provide opportunity.

comment opportunity An opportunity to communicate in which the child sees something novel or surprising and signals some kind of recognition. *See also* PoWRRS-Connect; provide opportunity.

communication continuum Description of developing communication, starting with forms that are reflexive, moving to pre-intentional preverbal behaviors, to intentional preverbal behaviors, and ultimately to symbolic forms.

communicative intentions Productions that are meant or interpreted to accomplish the following functional communication acts: requesting, commenting, protesting, acknowledging, and answering.

connect Element of PoWRRS-Connect that corresponds to adult interacting (or playing) with a child. *See also* PoWRRS-Connect.

dual focus Gaze from person to object, or object to person, or between two objects or two people. *See also* gaze; single focus; triadic focus.

families Caregivers and others living in the home or having regular contact with a child.

gaze Direction of the eyes. *See also* dual focus; single focus; triadic focus.

individuals with complex communication needs (CCNs) Description of children with disabilities including diverse, complex characteristics that interfere with connecting with others and the possibility of not using speech as a primary means of communication.

intentional communication Child productions of gaze, gestures, and/or vocalizations that are meant to communicate some type of functional act (e.g., requesting, commenting, protesting) to influence another person's behavior. Triadic gaze has been viewed as a clear signal of intentional communication, and as such, the hallmark of this developmental milestone.

potential level of performance   Level of skill or behavior at which the child can perform with assistance from others. *See also* actual level of performance.

PoWRRS-Connect   Acronym for the six-element protocol used in Triadic Gaze Intervention: *P*rovide *o*pportunity, *W*ait, *R*ecognize the child's communication attempt, *R*espond to child's communication attempt, *S*hape to a more sophisticated form, and *C*onnect/interact with the child. *See also* Triadic Gaze Intervention (TGI).

practitioners   Early intervention professionals who work with families and children. These professionals are sometimes referred to as clinicians or EI specialists, and include, but are not limited to, speech-language pathologists, occupational therapists, physical therapists, educators, early interventionists, and psychologists.

primary service provider (PSP)   The early intervention team member who is selected to directly interact with the family. This person represents the team and is the liaison between the team and the family. This person is also the one to visit children and families and provide guidance in delivery of intervention in the child's natural environment during the family's authentic routines.

preintentional communication   Child productions of gaze, gestures, and vocalizations that may be purposeful, yet not intentionally used to communicate.

prelinguistic forms   *See* preverbal communication behaviors.

preverbal communication behaviors   Nonverbal behaviors that occur prior to the production of first words, signs, or symbols, and include gaze, gestures, and vocalizations.

prompts   Verbal, visual, auditory, and/or tactile cues used to support a child's performance of a more sophisticated, conventional communication behavior. *See also* shape.

provide opportunity   Element of *Po*WRRS-Connect that corresponds to setting up a communication occasion designed to elicit a response from a child. Communication opportunities primarily consist of choice, request, and comment opportunities. *See also* choice opportunity; comment opportunity; PoWRRS-Connect; request opportunity.

purposeful behaviors   Child productions of preverbal behaviors that are not reflexive. They may be purposefully produced by the child but are not meant to influence the behavior of others. In this book, they are contrasted with intentional communication.

recognize   Element of PoW*R*RS-Connect that corresponds to the adult's effort to identify and interpret a child's communication attempt. *See also* PoWRRS-Connect.

reflexive behaviors   Child production of behaviors that are not purposeful or intentional. They reflect a physiological state (e.g., hunger, fatigue), for example, crying, fussing, squealing, and/or waving arms.

request opportunity   An opportunity to communicate where a child is offered an object or toy that requires an adult's help to obtain or operate, or the child is offered an opportunity to take a turn in a back-and-forth social exchange (e.g., singing songs). *See also* PoWRRS-Connect; provide opportunity.

respond   Element of PoWR*R*S-Connect that corresponds to the adult's response to a child's attempt to communicate. *See also* PoWRRS-Connect.

routines-based intervention Approach to early intervention where everyday activities in the natural environment serve as the context for working with families and children. *See also* authentic routines.

shape Element of PoWRRS-Connect that corresponds to assistance or support in the form of prompts that are provided by an adult to help a child successfully perform a behavior or task that is just beyond their capacity. *Scaffolding* is a term used among professionals to describe shaping. *See also* PoWRRS-Connect; prompts.

single focus Body orientation and gaze to a person or an object. *See also* dual focus; gaze; triadic focus.

symbolic communication Production of signs, spoken words, and/or icons or other symbolic representations or forms; can be used in augmentative and alternative communication.

TGI *see* Triadic Gaze Intervention.

triadic focus Three-point gaze that shifts back and forth between person, object, and person or object, person, and object. Hallmark of intentional communication. *See also* dual focus; gaze; single focus.

Triadic Gaze Intervention (TGI) A conceptual strategy that recognizes the importance of engagement and communication during the first year of life. The strategy focuses on helping families engage and communicate with their young children by recognizing their children's communication attempts and increasing their children's repertoire of conventional/recognizable preverbal behaviors. TGI is based on literature that describes early preverbal development that consists of gaze, gestural, and vocal behaviors that build the foundation for intentional communication (defined by triadic focus) and on to expanded communication of various forms (spoken words, signs, symbols). The TGI strategy is implemented in practice through the PoWRRS-Connect protocol. *See also* PoWRRS-Connect.

wait Element of PoWRRS-Connect that corresponds to the adult pausing long enough for the child to produce a communicative behavior. *See also* PoWRRS-Connect.

References

Adamson, L., Bakeman, R., Deckner, D., & Nelson, P. (2014). Interactions to conversations: The development of joint engagement during early childhood. *Child Development, 85*(3), 941–955.

Adamson, L., & Dimitrova, N. (2014). Joint attention and language development. In P. J. Brooks & V. Kempe (Eds.), *Encyclopedia of language development* (pp. 299–304). SAGE Reference. https://link-gale.com.offcampus.lib.washington.edu/apps/doc/CX6500800105/GVRL?u=wash_main&sid=GVRL&xid=9b9dd5e2

American Speech-Language-Hearing Association. (2008a). *Core knowledge and skills in early intervention speech-language pathology practice.* http://www.asha.org/policy

American Speech-Language-Hearing Association. (2008b). *Roles and responsibilities of speech-language pathologists in early intervention: Guidelines.* http://www.asha.org/policy

American Speech-Language-Hearing Association. (2008c). *Roles and responsibilities of speech-language pathologists in early intervention: Position statement.* http://www. asha.org/policy.

American Speech-Language-Hearing Association. (2008d). *Roles and responsibilities of speech-language pathologists in early intervention: Technical report.* http://www.asha. org/policy

Bakeman, R., & Adamson, L. (1984). Coordinating attention to people and objects in mother–infant and peer–infant interaction. *Child Development, 55*(4), 1278–1289.

Bakeman, R., & Brown, J. V. (1980). Early interaction: Consequences for social and mental development at three years. *Child Development, 51,* 437–447.

Bates, E., Camaioni, L., & Volterra, V. (1975). The acquisition of performatives prior to speech. *Merrill-Palmer Quarterly, 21*(3), 205–226.

Bayley, N. (2009). *Bayley-III: Bayley Scales of Infant and Toddler Development.* Pearson.

Beukelman, D. R., & Light, J. C. (2020). *Augmentative & alternative communication: Supporting children & adults with complex communication needs* (5th ed.). Paul H. Brookes Publishing Co.

Beukelman, D. R., & Mirenda, P. (2005). *Augmentative & alternative communication: Supporting children & adults with complex communication needs* (3rd ed.). Paul H. Brookes Publishing Co.

Beukelman, D. R., & Mirenda, P. (2013). *Augmentative & alternative communication: Supporting children & adults with complex communication needs* (4th ed.). Paul H. Brookes Publishing Co.

Beuker, K., Rommelse, N., Donders, R., & Buitelaar, J. (2013). Development of early communication skills in the first two years of life. *Infant Behavior and Development, 36*(1), 71–83.

Brady, N., Fleming, K., Thiemann-Bourke, K., Olswang, L., Dowden, P., & Saunders, M. (2012). Development of the Communication Complexity Scale. *American Journal of Speech-Language Pathology, 21,* 16–28.

Brady, N. C., & Warren, S. F. (2003). Language interventions for children with mental retardation. *International Review of Research in Mental Retardation, 27,* 231–254.

Brazelton, T. B. (1982). Joint regulation of neonate-parent behavior. In E. Z. Tronick (Ed.), *Social interchange in infancy: Affect, cognition, and communication* (pp. 7–22). University Park Press.

Brazelton, T. B. (1988). Importance of early intervention. In E. Hibbs (Ed.), *Children and families: Studies in prevention and intervention* (pp. 107–120). International University Press.

Brazelton, T. B. (1992). *Touchpoints: Emotional and behavioral development.* Addison-Wesley.

Brown, J., & Woods, J. (2015). Effects of a triadic parent-implemented home-based communication intervention for toddlers. *Journal of Early Intervention, 37,* 44–68.

Bruder, M. B. (2000). Family-centered early intervention: Clarifying our values for the new millennium. *Topics in Early Childhood Special Education, 20*(2), 105–115.

Bruner, J. (1982). The organization of action and the nature of the adult–infant transaction. In E. Z. Tronick (Ed.), *Social interchange in infancy: Affect, cognition, and communication* (pp. 23–35). University Park Press.

Bruner, J. (1983). *Child's talk: Learning to use language.* Norton.

Bruner, J. S. (1999). The intentionality of referring. In P. D. Zelazo, J. W. Astington, & D. R. Olson (Eds.), *Developing theories of intention* (pp. 329–339). Lawrence Erlbaum.

Campbell, P., Sawyer, B., & Muhlenhaupt, M. (2009). The meaning of natural environments for parents and professionals. *Infants and Young Children, 22,* 264–278.

Carpenter, R. L., Mastergeorge, A. M., & Coggins, T. E. (1983). The acquisition of communicative intentions in infants eight to fifteen months of age. *Language and Speech, 26*, 101–116.

Coggins, T. E., & Carpenter, R. L. (1981). The Communicative Intention Inventory: A system for observing and coding children's early intentional communication. *Applied Psycholinguistics, 2*, 235–251.

Cripe, J. W., & Venn, M. L. (1997). Family-guided routines for early intervention services. *Young Exceptional Children, 1*(1), 18–26.

Division for Early Childhood. (2014). *DEC recommended practices in early intervention/early childhood special education 2014.* http://www.dec-sped.org/recommendedpractices

Dowden, P., & Cook, A. M. (2012). Improving communicative competence through alternative selection methods. In S. Johnston, J. Reichle, K. Feeley, & J. Jones (Eds.), *Augmentative and alternative communication strategies for individuals with severe disabilities* (pp. 81–117). Paul H. Brookes Publishing Co.

Dunst, C. J., Hamby, D., Trivette, C. M., Raab, M., & Bruder, M. B. (2000). Everyday family and community life and children's naturally occurring learning opportunities. *Journal of Early Intervention, 23*, 151–164.

Early Childhood Technical Assistance Center (ECTA). (2014). *Integrating child and family outcomes into the individualized family service plan (IFSP) process.* https://ectacenter.org/eco/assets/pdfs/IFSP-OutcomesFlow Chart.pdf

Early Childhood Technical Assistance Center. (2015, March 4). *States' and territories' definitions of/criteria for IDEA Part C eligibility.* https://ectacenter.org/~pdfs/topics/earlyid/partc_elig_table.pdf

Early Childhood Technical Assistance Center. (2021, February 25). *Outcomes: Child outcomes.* https://ectacenter.org/eco/pages/childoutcomes.asp

Evidence-Based International Early Intervention Office (EIEIO). (n.d.). *EIEIO and the Routines Based Model.* http://eieio.ua.edu/routines-based-model.html

Feuerstein, J., & Olswang, L. (2020). A randomized controlled trial investigating online training for prelinguistic communication. *Journal of Speech, Language, and Hearing Research, 63*, 827–833.

Feuerstein, J., Olswang, L., Greenslade, K., Dowden, P., Pinder, G. L., & Madden, J. (2018). Implementation research: Embracing practitioners' views. *Journal of Speech, Language, and Hearing Research, 61*, 645–657.

Feuerstein, J., Olswang, L., Greenslade, K., Pinder, G. L., Dowden, P., & Madden, J. (2017). Moving triadic gaze intervention into practice: Measuring clinician attitude and implementation fidelity. *Journal of Speech, Language, and Hearing Research, 60*(5), 1285–1298.

Feuerstein, R., Rand, Y., & Hoffman, M. (1979). *The dynamic assessment of retarded performers: The learning potential assessment device, theory, instruments, and techniques.* Scott Foresman.

Fiese, B., & Sameroff, A. (1989). Family context in pediatric psychology: A transactional perspective. *Journal of Pediatric Psychology, 14*(2), 293–314.

Gates, M. (2019). *The moment of lift: How empowering women changes the world.* Flatiron Books.

Girolametto, L. (1988). Improving the social-conversational skills of developmentally delayed children: An intervention study. *Journal of Speech and Hearing Disorders, 53*, 156–167.

Guralnick, M. J. (2001). A developmental systems model for early intervention. *Infants & Young Children, 14*(2), 1–18.

Halle, J., Brady, N., & Drasgow, E. (2004). Enhancing socially adaptive communicative repairs of beginning communicators with disabilities. *American Journal of Speech-Language Pathology, 13*(1), 43–54.

Hanft, B. E., Rush, D. D., & Shelden, M. L. (2004). *Coaching families and colleagues in early childhood.* Paul H. Brookes Publishing Co.

Hanft, B. E., Rush, D. D., & Shelden, M. L. (2020). *Coaching families and colleagues in early childhood* (2nd ed.). Paul H. Brookes Publishing Co.

Hebbeler, K., Spiker, D., Bailey, D., Scarborough, A., Mallik, S., Simeonsson, R., Singer, M., & Nelson, L. (2007). *Early intervention for infants & toddlers with disabilities and their families: Participants, services, and outcomes* (Final report of the National Early Intervention Longitudinal Study). https://www.sri.com/sites/default/files/publications/neils_finalreport_200702.pdf

Iacono, T. (2014). What it means to have complex communication needs. *Research and Practice in Intellectual and Developmental Disabilities, 1*(1), 82–85. doi:10.1080/23297018.2014.908814

Iacono, T., Carter, M., & Hook, J. (1998). Identification of intentional communication in students with severe and multiple disabilities. *Augmentative and Alternative Communication, 14*(2), 102–114.

Individuals with Disabilities Education Act. (2001). Early Intervention Program for Infants and Toddlers With Disabilities. 76 C.F.R § 300, 303. https://www.govinfo.gov/content/pkg/FR-2011-09-28/pdf/2011-22783.pdf

Individuals with Disabilities Education Improvement Act (IDEA) of 2004, PL 108-446, 20 U.S.C. §§ 1400 *et seq.*

Kaiser, A., & Roberts, M. (2013). Parent-implemented Enhanced Milieu Teaching with preschool children with intellectual disabilities. *Journal of Speech, Language & Hearing Association, 56*, 295–309.

Kasari, C., Freeman, S. F. N., & Paparella, T. (2001). Early intervention in autism: Joint attention and symbolic play. *International Review of Research in Mental Retardation, 23*, 207–237.

Kelly, J. F., Zuckerman, T., & Rosenblatt, S. (2008). Promoting first relationships: A relationship-focused early intervention approach. *Infants & Young Children, 21*(4), 285–295.

King, G., Strachan, D., Tucker, M., Duwyn, B., Desserud, S., & Shillington, B. (2009). The application of a transdisciplinary model for early intervention services. *Infants & Young Children, 22*(3), 211–223.

Locke, J. (1993). *The child's path to spoken language.* Harvard University Press.

McCathren, R., & Warren, S. F. (1996). Prelinguistic predictors of later language development. In K. N. Cole, P. S. Dale, & D. J. Thal (Eds.), *Communication and language intervention series: Assessment of communication and language* (Vol. 6, pp. 57–75). Paul H. Brookes Publishing Co.

McWilliam, R. A. (2010a). *Routines-based early intervention.* Paul H. Brookes Publishing Co.

McWilliam, R. A. (Ed.). (2010b). Assessing families' needs with the routines-based interview. In *Working with families of young children with special needs* (pp. 27–59). Guilford.

Mundy, P., & Newell, L. (2007). Attention, joint attention, and social cognition. *Current Directions in Psychological Science, 16,* 269–274. [PubMed: 19343102]

Mundy, P., Sigman, M., & Kasari, C. (1990). A longitudinal study of joint attention and language development in autistic children. *Journal of Autism and Developmental Disorders, 20*(1), 115–128.

Murray, L., & Trevarthen, C. (1986). The infant's role in mother–infant communication. *Journal of Child Language, 4*(1), 1–22.

National Research Council & Institute of Medicine, Committee on Integrating the Science of Early Childhood Development. (2000). In J. P. Shonkoff & D. A. Phillips (Eds.), *Executive summary* (p. 7). National Academies Press.

Nursing Child Assessment Satellite Training (NCAST), University of Washington School of Nursing. (n.d.). *The six states of consciousness* [course handout].

Office of Special Education Programs. (2019). *OSEP indicators and outcomes.* https://connectmodules.dec-sped.org/wp-content/uploads/2019/03/CONNECT-M1-OSEP-SPP-APR.pdf

Olswang, L., Dowden, P., Feuerstein, J., Greenslade, K., Pinder, G. L., & Fleming, K. (2014). Triadic gaze intervention for young children with physical disabilities. *Journal of Speech-Language, and Hearing Research, 57,* 1740–1753.

Olswang, L., Feuerstein, J., Pinder, G. L., & Dowden, P. (2013). Validating dynamic assessment of triadic gaze for young children with severe disabilities. *American Journal of Speech-Language Pathology, 22,* 449–462.

Olswang, L., & Pinder, G. L. (1995). Preverbal functional communication and the role of object play in children with cerebral palsy. *Infant-Toddler Intervention, 5,* 277–300.

Olswang, L., Pinder, G. L., & Hanson, R. (2006). Communication in young children with motor impairments: Teaching caregivers to teach. *Seminars in Speech and Language, 27,* 199–214.

Paparella, T., & Kasari, C. (2004). Joint attention skills and language development in special needs populations: Translating research to practice. *Infants and Young Children, 17*(3), 269–280.

Paul, D., & Roth, F. (2011). Guiding principles and clinical applications for speech-language pathology practice in early intervention. *Language, Speech, and Hearing Services in Schools, 42,* 320–330.

Pinder, G. L., & Olswang, L. (1995). Development of communicative intent in young children with cerebral palsy: A treatment efficacy study. *Infant-Toddler Intervention, 5,* 51–69.

Pinder, G. L., Olswang, L., & Coggins, K. (1993). The development of communicative intent in a physically disabled child. *Infant-Toddler Intervention, 3,* 1–17.

Prizant, B. M., Wetherby, A. M., Rubin, E., Laurent, A. C., & Rydell, P. (2006). *The SCERTS® model: A comprehensive educational approach for children with autism spectrum disorders.* Paul H. Brookes Publishing Co.

Roman-Lantzy, C. (2018). *Cortical visual impairment: An approach to assessment and intervention* (2nd ed.). American Foundation for the Blind.

Rossetti, L. M. (2006). *The Rossetti Infant-Toddler Language Scale.* LinguiSystems.

Rush, D., & Shelden, M. L. (2011). *The early childhood coaching handbook.* Paul H. Brookes Publishing Co.

Rush, D., & Shelden, M. L. (2020). *The early childhood coaching handbook* (2nd ed.). Paul H. Brookes Publishing Co.

Salisbury, C., Woods, J., Snyder, P., Moddelmog, K., Mawdsley, H., Romano, M., & Windsor, K. (2018). Caregiver and provider experiences with coaching and embedded intervention. *Topics in Early Childhood Special Education, 38*(1), 17–29.

Salley B., Brady N. C., Hoffman, L., & Fleming, K. (2019). Preverbal communication complexity in infants. *Infancy, 25,* 4–21.

Sameroff, A. (1987). The social context of development. In N. Eisenberg (Ed.), *Contemporary topics in developmental psychology* (pp. 273–291). Wiley.

Sameroff, A. J., & Fiese, B. H. (1990). Transactional regulation and early intervention. In S. J. Meisels & J. P. Shonkoff (Eds.), *Early intervention: A handbook of theory, practice and analysis* (pp. 119–149). Cambridge University Press.

Sandall, S. R., Hemmeter, M. L., Smith, B. J., & McLean, M. E. (2005). *DEC recommended practices: A comprehensive guide for practical application in early intervention/early childhood special education.* Division for Early Childhood, Council for Exceptional Children.

Shelden, M., & Rush, D. (2013). *The early intervention teaming handbook: The primary service provider approach.* Paul H. Brookes Publishing Co.

Sigafoos, J., & Mirenda, P. (2002). Strengthening communication behaviors for gaining access to desired items and activities. In J. Reichle, D. Beukelman, & J. Light (Eds.), *Exemplary practices for beginning communicators: Implications for AAC* (pp. 123–156). Paul H. Brookes Publishing Co.

Tannock, R., Girolametto, L., & Siegel, L. (1992). Language intervention with children who have developmental delays: Effects of an interactive approach. *American Journal of Mental Retardation, 97,* 145–160.

Thomasello, M. (1999). Having intentions, understanding intentions, and understanding communicative intentions. In P. D. Zelazo & J. Wilded (Eds.), *Developing theories of intention: Social understanding and self-control* (pp. 63–75). Lawrence Erlbaum.

Trevarthen, C., & Aitken, K. (2001). Infant intersubjectivity: Research, theory, and clinical applications. *Journal of Child Psychology and Psychiatry, 42*(1), 3–48.

Trevarthen, C., & Hubley, P. (1978). Secondary intersubjectivity: Confidence, confiding, and acts of meaning in the first year. In A. Lock (Ed.), *Action, gesture and symbol: The emergence of language* (pp. 183–229). Academic Press.

Voress, J., Maddox, T., & Hammill, D. (2012). *Developmental Assessment of Young Children–Second Edition* (DAYC-2). PRO-ED.

Warren, S. F., Bredin-Oja, S. L., Fairchild, M. A., Finestack, L. H., Fey, M. E., & Brady, N. C. (2006). Responsivity education/prelinguistic milieu teaching. In R. J. McCauley, M. E. Fey, & R. Gillam (Eds.), *Communication and language intervention series: Treatment of language disorders in children,* (2nd ed., pp. 47–75). Paul H. Brookes Publishing Co.

Wilcox, M., & Woods, J. (2011). Participation as a basis for developing, early intervention outcomes. *Language, Speech, and Hearing Services in Schools, 42,* 365–378.

Windsor, K., Woods, J., Kaiser, A., Snyder, P., & Salisbury, C. (2019). Caregiver-implemented intervention for communication and motor outcomes for infants and toddlers. *Topics in Early Childhood Special Education, 39*(2), 73–87.

Woods, J. (2005). *Family-guided routines-based intervention project.* Florida State University, Department of Communication Disorders.

Woods, J., Kashinath, S., & Goldstein, H. (2004). Effects of embedding caregiver implementation teaching strategies in daily routines in children's communication outcomes. *Journal of Early Intervention, 26,* 175–193.

Woods, J. J., & Wetherby, A. M. (2003). Early identification of and intervention for infants and toddlers who are at risk for autism spectrum disorder. *Language, Speech & Hearing Services in the Schools, 34*(3), 180–193.

Yoder, P. J., & Warren, S. F. (1993). Can developmentally delayed children's language development be enhanced through prelinguistic intervention? In A. P. Kaiser & D. B. Gray (Eds.), *Enhancing children's communication: Research foundations for intervention* (Vol. 2, pp. 35–61). Paul H. Brookes Publishing Co.

Yoder, P. J., & Warren, S. F. (2002). Effects of prelinguistic milieu teaching and parent responsivity education on dyads involving children with intellectual disabilities. *Journal of Speech, Language, Hearing Research, 45,* 1158–1174.

Zimmerman, I., Steiner, V., & Pond, R. (2011). *Preschool Language Scales* (5th ed.). Pearson.

Index

References to tables and figures are indicated with a *t*, and *f*, respectively